SpringerBriefs in Crim

For further volumes:
http://www.springer.com/series/10159

David N. Khey • John Stogner • Bryan Lee Miller

Emerging Trends in Drug Use and Distribution

Volume 12

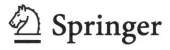 Springer

David N. Khey
Department of Criminal Justice
Loyola University New Orleans
New Orleans
Louisiana
USA

Bryan Lee Miller
Dept of Criminal Justice and Criminology
Georgia Southern University
Statesboro
Georgia
USA

John Stogner
Dept. of Criminal Justice
University of North Carolina Charlotte
Charlotte
USA

ISSN 2192-8533   ISSN 2192-8541 (electronic)
ISBN 978-3-319-03574-1   ISBN 978-3-319-03575-8 (eBook)
DOI 10.1007/978-3-319-03575-8
Springer Cham Heidelberg New York Dordrecht London

Library of Congress Control Number: 2013954904

Printed on acid-free paper

Springer is part of Springer Science+Business Media (www.springer.com)

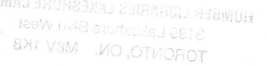

Preface

Cannabinoids are the crisis of the decade

Evren et al. 2013

Concerns over the increased use of emerging drugs—especially among teenagers—have captured the attention of the media, legislatures, and local communities. However, there has been a great deal of misinformation, sensationalistic journalism, and uncertainty in regards to these sorts of substances. Policy-makers have recently erred on the side of caution by taking strides to ban these substances shortly after a first mention of them in the headlines. Many public health experts seemingly fail to understand the broader patterns of emerging drug use, particularly in context of a wealth of previous cases and patterns seen over the last century. With the increasing number of current cases requiring governmental and public health intervention, we wish to arm decision-makers with a comprehensive guide on emerging drugs to make informed decisions. We hope that they will begin to see the emergence of new psychoactive drugs not as unique overwhelming crises, but as patterned events that may be managed. For students, researchers, and parents, we wish to provide a balanced source of information on this topic; but, most importantly, we wish to dispel the misconceptions and shine light on actualized problems to give us a clear understanding of the issues pertaining to emerging drugs.

Contents

1 New Trends in Psychoactive Drug Use 1
  1.1 Introduction 1
  1.2 Defining Emerging Drugs 3
  1.3 Sources of Emerging Drugs 5
  1.4 General Patterns of Use 6
  1.5 Public Health Concerns 7
  1.6 Divergence from Federal Guidance and Law 9
  1.7 Setting the Tone 10
  References 10

2 Emerging Drugs, Today Versus Yesteryear 13
  2.1 Partitioning Recreational Drugs from Medicine 13
    2.1.1 Absinthe 14
    2.1.2 LSD 18
    2.1.3 Quaalude 21
    2.1.4 MDMA, Ketamine, and GHB 23
  2.2 Drug Scares and the Media 25
  2.3 Current Trends 26
    2.3.1 Newly Synthesized Analogues 26
    2.3.2 New to Us—Botanicals 28
    2.3.3 New Tricks for Old Drugs 29
  2.4 Connecting the Past to the Present 30
  References 31

**3 Emerging Drug Trade and Use: Manufacturing, Marketing,
and Understanding Novel Highs** 33
  3.1 The Shadow Industry Profiting from Emerging Drug Use 33
    3.1.1 Drug Development and the Regulate and Reformulate
Game 35
    3.1.2 Distribution and International Issues 37
  3.2 The Sale and Marketing of Novel Drugs 38
    3.2.1 Over the Counter Retail Sales 38

3.2.2 Street Dealers and Black Market Distribution 39
3.2.3 Online Sales 40
3.3 The Role of the Internet in the Spread of Emerging Drugs 42
3.4 Explaining Emerging Drug Use 43
3.4.1 Traditional Explanations of Drug Use 44
3.4.2 Emerging Drugs as Replacements for Banned Substances . . . 46
3.4.3 Emerging Drug Use as a Deviant Social Milestone 47
References 48

4 Case Studies of Emerging Drugs: Salvia, Bath Salts,
and Bromo-DragonFly 53
4.1 Case Study 1: *Salvia divinorum* 53
4.1.1 Historic Use of Salvia 54
4.1.2 Modern Salvia Use 54
4.1.3 Media Coverage and Regulation of Salvia 55
4.1.4 The Scope of Salvia Use 56
4.1.5 Salvia: An Internet Phenomenon? 58
4.1.6 Typology of Salvia Users 59
4.1.7 Lessons from Salvia Use in the USA 61
4.2 Case Study 2: Synthetic Stimulants Called "Bath Salts" 61
4.2.1 Bath Salts and the Body 62
4.2.2 The Emergence of Bath Salt Use 63
4.2.3 US Media and Cultural Panics Linked to Bath Salt Use 65
4.2.4 Regulation of Bath Salts and Results 66
4.2.5 Lessons from Bath Salts and the Future 67
4.3 Case Study 3: Bromo-DragonFly, a Powerful Hallucinogen 68
References 70

5 What Is Being Done About Emerging Drugs? 75
5.1 The Controlled Substances Act 75
5.1.1 Emergency Scheduling Powers 76
5.1.2 Controlled Substance Analogues 77
5.1.3 Food and Drug Administration 78
5.2 A Move Away from the CSA 79
5.2.1 State-Level Medicalization of Marijuana 80
5.2.2 Salvia divinorum, Kratom, and other State Level Bans 80
5.3 Synthetic Cannabinoids, Bath Salts, and the Synthetic
Drug Abuse Prevention Act of 2012 83
5.4 International Regulations of Emerging Drugs 84
5.5 Law Enforcement and Interdiction 84
5.6 Prosecuting Emerging Drug Cases 87
5.7 Crime Lab and Drug Testing 88
5.8 Emerging Drug Prevention 89
5.9 Future Directions 90
References 92

Index 95

Chapter 1
New Trends in Psychoactive Drug Use

Over the past two decades in particular, there has been increasing concern over a subset of psychoactive substances new on the drug scene. While some have received a substantial amount of media coverage in recent years, many of these substances are unheard of by the vast populous; in fact, only a niche group of drug users may know of their existence previous to their eventual exposure to the public. There is, however, a good base for understanding these emerging drugs as presented in this chapter. A framework is presented to better grapple with emerging drug trends given this knowledge base. This provides a solid foundation to expand on previous research while minimizing the temptation of including anecdotal and circumstantial evidence when drawing conclusions on emerging drug trends.

1.1 Introduction

To say the least, emerging drugs have captured a share of media headlines in recent years. The litany of stories has ranged from reports of celebrity use and reviews of legal changes to fear-mongering pieces about epidemic use among teenagers and the drugs' close connections with criminal activity and bizarre behavior. Members of mainstream America seem to know of these drugs only as a result of a handful of over-sensationalized cases in the media. A perfect case in point was the intense media interest in the videotape depicting popular musician Miley Cyrus "tripping out" after smoking the plant *Salvia divinorum* (Detrick 2010). The coverage of this leaked clip rapidly elevated the awareness of salvia among the American public, as the untimely death of Brett Chidester had years before (Griffin et al. 2008). In 2006, the 17-year-old took his own life, and salvia use was officially listed on the death certificate as a contributing cause of death. Or take the case of award-winning actress Demi Moore: After experiencing complications and convulsions attributed to smoking synthetic cannabinoids, she was rushed to the hospital and treated for drug poisoning. As a result, reports of cannabinoid issues increased manyfold across the nation and media consumers were exposed to the "wild dangers" of a new and emerging drug trend (Dillon 2012). Perhaps receiving the most attention was the incredible story of a drug-crazed, zombie-like attack on an unsuspecting Florida man in 2012. Despite

D. N. Khey et al., *Emerging Trends in Drug Use and Distribution*,
SpringerBriefs in Criminology 12, DOI 10.1007/978-3-319-03575-8_1,
© Springer International Publishing Switzerland 2014

the subsequent confirmation of the lack of synthetic cathinones in Rudy Eugene's system at the time of his violent and cannibalistic attack on Ronald Poppo in southern Florida (Hiaasen and Green 2012), many Americans still associate bath salts with cannibalism as a result of the extensive media coverage and gross misreporting of the incident.

Though the fear and anxieties related to new and emerging drugs seem to be based on a few isolated incidents and inaccurate information, this certainly does not mean that those concerns are inappropriate. Quite to the contrary, and as the following chapters will demonstrate, some of the recently emerging drugs represent a clear threat to public health and should be the focus of regulation and intense concerted effort of emergency medicine, treatment professionals, law enforcement (particularly as related to interdiction), and customs and postal inspectors. However, in order to best manage the appearance of new drug trends and new substances, a better and more analytic approach to the emerging drug problem must be undertaken. Rather than react with panic and engage in knee-jerk reactions, an informed society should focus on gathering facts about novel substances' pharmacology, effects, use patterns, distribution, and risk-potential. Importantly, an educated society should also consider the social dynamics that led to the drugs' emergence. Doing so will give us a window into an emerging drug's potential for problematic and/or dangerous use. For example, if we know that a new substance is being primarily used in the club scene, there may be potential for this substance to be combined with other drugs (ecstasy, LSD, and perhaps alcohol)—which may lead to unintended consequences. Further, policymakers should avoid outright bans on these substances until they explore the full ramifications of these actions. This includes the effect of regulation on law enforcement (such as cost and distraction from larger concerns), the potential for "legal high" manufacturers to replace a banned substance with a more dangerous or addicting unregulated formulation of the drug, and whether users will revert to more dangerous street drugs. There are also various other tools available to legislatures, public health and justice professionals, and others involved to mitigate the problems of novel substances, minimize use (particularly problem use), and optimize public resources available to address these problems. Alternative approaches to an immediate outright ban also allow more latitude to researchers in investigating potential therapeutic agents and reduces the likelihood that these substances will be mired in the typical stigma attached to "illicit drugs," "drugs of abuse," or "illegal drugs."

The following chapters offer insight into the emerging drug phenomenon in an attempt to assist readers in reaching valid conclusions and inspire thoughtful research in the area. They stress that while many psychoactive substances are new to recreational use (including most of those that serve as examples within the text), the phenomenon of emerging drugs is not. Modern societies have struggled to manage numerous substances hyped as the "next scary drug" for many decades. Chapter 2 offers several examples of the management of historical emerging drug "threats" and outlines how some of these drugs became a permanent part of today's drug landscape while others fell from popular use. The chapter then introduces some prominent contemporary emerging drug issues and makes clear the similarities of past and present emerging drug narratives. By presenting the information in this way, we emphasize that it is not so much the drugs themselves that are critically important relative to the societal and cultural factors that shape these narratives. Readers should utilize this balanced and historically grounded approach to augment the recent focus on the chemical specifics of these drugs. In particular, understanding the process through which new drugs are developed, introduced, marketed, promoted, reported on, regulated, and become the subject of law enforcement and regulatory efforts will enhance readers' understanding related to all new drugs and serve them better than a focus on a single drug's chemical composition. The patterns seen in today's emerging drugs repeat those of historic emerging drugs and will likely be repeated in the future with new substances and new forms of existing drugs. As a result, understanding the emergence of these drugs will help readers predict the evolution in the use of new drugs reaching the market in future.

1.2 Defining Emerging Drugs

At present, there seems to be as much inconsistency with labeling and categorizing emerging drugs as there is with regulating and reacting to the substances. Determining the appropriate nomenclature and taxonomy for these substances that have only recently been used for recreational purposes is tricky in that these drugs vary in terms of their origin, psychoactive effects, legality, and distribution. Unlike the traditional categorizations of drugs as stimulants, depressants, hallucinogens, and so forth, each of these substances are *evolving in use* in a similar way rather than sharing a cluster of psychological and physiological effects. However, their collective grouping serves a clear purpose. They may be linked to similar portions of a "shadow industry" and their manufacturers may utilize similar practices to skirt the law and reach consumers. Even law enforcement and public health officials have limited knowledge of their pharmacological effects and may think of each of these substances as "one of those new drugs." With evolution being their unifying trait, determining which substances should be placed in this framework is challenging in that several features of a drug itself and its use patterns may be actively changing. This could include new formulations, new marketing techniques, altered routes of administration, or other changes.

In recent years, the term "legal highs" was employed to describe several of the substances that we consider emerging drugs, particularly by the media; this term also carried over to several recent academic studies (e.g., Brandt et al. 2010; Arunotayanun and Gibbons 2012; Davies et al. 2010). As Corazza et al. (2012) point out, it is inappropriate to apply the "legal" label since a substance's legality may change soon after its emergence and legal status can vary across jurisdictions. Further, many substances may initially exist in a legal "gray area" in that their legality or illegality may be contingent on an administrative ruling that determines if a substance in question is similar enough to a currently banned substance to be considered an analogue; that is, many nations have created laws to regulate substances which are chemically and functionally related to an existing controlled substance. Additionally, the "legal high" label may also lead potential users to continue to infer that the substance remains legal after a ban (Singleton et al. in press). Academics have also pointed out that "high" may be more of a marketing ploy than an accurate description of a product's actual effects. They suggest that the word is included to reinforce perceptions that the drug's effects are pleasurable (Corazza et al. 2012). In fact, users of some substances may label the effects as something other than a "high." Those that have experimented with certain drugs might avoid this language (Khey et al. 2008).

The terms "synthetic legal intoxicating drugs (SLIDs)," "designer drugs," and "synthetic drugs" are also frequently used in academic literature (e.g., Jerry et al. 2012; Vardakou et al. 2011). We offer similar objections to the "legal" portion of the SLIDs term as noted previously for "legal highs." These descriptions are moreover problematic in that they exclude products that have natural (e.g., botanical) origins. The category should include plant-based drugs that are emerging onto the drug scene (such as *S. divinorum* and kratom); the "synthetic" moniker implies only synthesized compounds can or should be included. While these labels may be appropriate to use in discussions of subgroups of emerging drugs such as those marketed as "bath salts," it is preferable to use a more inclusive term for the entire group.

Not surprisingly, the underground even has its own accepted vernacular for emerging drugs. The seemingly generic term "research chemicals" appears to be an underground code for a broad range of these substances (see Chap. 2 for more details) and seems to be an equivalent to the terms SLIDs, designer drugs, or synthetic drugs described above. That is, the term tends to describe synthetic or semi-synthetic products that are available in the underground marketplace. Other underground terms such as "botanicals" or "ethnobotanicals" reflect some of the plant or plant-based products being used recreationally. If you look intently, one can find hundreds of psychoactive research chemicals and botanicals that are unlikely to emerge as recreational drugs of choice or as public health threats. Most are obscure substances and natural products that few users or law enforcement will ever come across, at least knowingly.

Miller et al. (2013) define the term "novel drug" as either a newly discovered recreational substance or an existing substance that has only recently been used for recreational purposes. Corazza et al. (2012) offer a similar definition for their term, "novel psychoactive drug (NPD)." While we appreciate each of these classifications, we have come to the conclusion that the term "emerging drugs" best fits the wide range of issues public health experts face in regard to these more obscure substances. "Emerging drugs" incorporates every substance that meets the Miller et al. (2013) and Corazza et al.'s (2012) criteria; it also is purposefully intended to be more comprehensive and inclusive. It implies that categorization is based on a drugs' new presence in social setting rather than a new presence in laboratory. Also, and importantly, it does not matter if this laboratory is a legitimate pharmaceutical research facility, if it exists in a rogue underground chemist's basement, or if a foreign laboratory or chemical manufacturing facility is skirting laws or operating in the gray area afforded by current drug legislation; the emphasis is focused on recreational use patterns within a defined geography. As noted previously, the most distinguishing characteristic of these drugs is change. We include drugs that are newly created, newly utilized for recreational purposes, and those finding themselves newly popular, but also include substances that are experiencing any other important change in their use. Therefore, a new route of drug administration would qualify as this change may substantially increase a drug's potency and user experience. Examples of current emerging drugs include those marketed as bath salts, synthetic cannabinoids, *S. divinorum*, purple drank, butane-extracted hash oil (BHO), Bromo-DragonFly, Euphoria, TMFPP, and an array of other similar products.

1.3   Sources of Emerging Drugs

Though emerging drugs may reach consumers in a variety of ways, many of today's emerging drugs owe their origins to a shadow industry that produces and distributes products intended to circumvent regulation and taxation. For example, many manufacturers, believed to operate primarily out of China, India, Pakistan, and other developing countries (Sumnall et al. 2011; National Drug Intelligence Center 2011), profit from producing and selling packages of substances that promise euphoria or other pleasurable psychoactive effects without legal ramifications. Though several products labeled as "legal highs" include illicit compounds (Ayres and Bond 2012) and have previously avoided inspection due to "not for human consumption" labels (Fass et al. 2012), this characterization may have led consumers to misperceive that the products are manufactured and evaluated with the same safety standards as other store-bought products. Essentially, this deception results in even less oversight than "dietary supplements" on the market, which must bear the message: "This statement has not been evaluated by the Food and Drug Administration (FDA). This product is not intended to diagnose, treat, cure, or prevent any disease" (Food and Drug Administration 2013). The merchandise produced by this shadow industry typically reaches the end consumer via tobacco outlets, head shops, tattoo parlors, gas stations, convenience stores, and the Internet prior to bans (Dargan et al. 2010; Jerry et al. 2012), and via street dealers and the Internet after bans (Winstock et al. 2010). The role of the shadow industry in expanding emerging drug use is covered in more detail in Chap. 3.

Other emerging drugs may involve what can be referred to as "kitchen chemistry," where a new psychoactive substance is formulated from precursor chemicals, a compound is chemically manipulated into a more powerful psychoactive form, or a drug is altered so that it may be taken in a new way. The emergence of new forms of kitchen chemistry may be linked to an increasingly educated drug-using population that has access to online guides and forums that coach their drug preparations (Cone 2006). It is more likely, however, that individuals who produce these sorts of substances have an advanced working knowledge of chemistry and have access to sophisticated instrumentation to produce a lab-quality product. Furthermore, some psychoactive substances have a legitimate purpose in the scientific research community, perhaps even those made popular by clandestine laboratories. They may become emerging drugs if their psychoactivity is newly discovered among recreational drug users, and/or if they become diverted from legitimate source. The shadow industry may also partition and package research chemicals in a form that is more easily accessed by the public. A long-lasting hallucinogen, Bromo-DragonFly, is an excellent example of a research chemical that is an emerging drug and is explored as a case study in Chap. 4.

1.4   General Patterns of Use

While we group emerging drugs based, in part, on their novelty and marketing practices, their general patterns of use are largely divergent. In many respects, use patterns of novel drugs resemble that of their respective "traditional" analogues. For example, the emerging drugs that can best be classified as hallucinogens seem to follow the patterns of LSD and other psychedelics; all of these substances are rarely used habitually and users rarely report dependence. The emerging drugs with stimulant properties, however, have been linked with psychological dependence and are more likely to be used repetitively and impulsively like many drugs in that class. Just like users of their traditional analogues (e.g., methamphetamine or cocaine), synthetic cathinone users have been reported to "binge" or "run" on the substance (Dybdal-Hargreaves et al. 2013). That is, they continue to administer additional doses of the drug during the high in order to intensify, maintain, and perpetuate the experience. As is the case for traditional stimulants, users may experience a severe crash after taking the drug. Another example of a group of emerging drugs that mirror their analogues can be found with the synthetic cannabinoids and cannabis products. These products may be used in a way similar to smoked marijuana, but not completely. It seems that the previous lack of regulation of synthetic cannabinoids and the former inability to be detected on drug tests were the leading rationales for use (Vandrey et al. 2012). Thus, this family of drugs may have served more as a substitute for marijuana as opposed to being the primary drug users craved. That is, they were likely seen as a less desirable and more costly alternative to marijuana, but used due to the occasional challenges with obtaining marijuana and, in particular, the initial lack of formal consequences.

Our awareness of novel drug use is somewhat confined to a small segment of the population, namely older adolescents and young adults. Existing research has focused on use within these groups as they are the predominate users of illicit substances in general. This assumption (that these age groups are the primary users of emerging drugs) seems to be supported by anecdotal evidence, case reports, and media coverage. Scientific data from national surveys that assess the prevalence of a variety of drugs (such as the NSDUH) seem to confirm that early childhood or late adult use of emerging drugs is rare in the United States and abroad. However, there seems to be a significant number of individuals in either high school or in their early adult years that experiment with emerging drugs, especially when they are marketed as "legal highs" or "legal" forms of popular illicit substances such as marijuana, cocaine, methamphetamines, or ecstasy. Many studies find that over 10 % of American high school and college students have used an emerging drug at least once (Johnston et al. 2013; Stogner and Miller 2013). Yet, it appears that very few users progress to habitual use of these substances. This suggests that a variety of emerging drugs have low continuance rates (e.g., the rate of users that progress to moderate to chronic use) and are not a key component of many young people's lives. On the other hand, these products have gained an underground relevance guaranteeing their survival far into the future in some form despite attempts to regulate them. To help understand these patterns, there are numerous theoretical explanations of emerging drug use that are explored in Chap. 3.

1.5 Public Health Concerns

While the emerging drug phenomenon is often primarily viewed as a legal issue to be handled by the legislature, courts, and law enforcement, its most substantial impact is likely to be on the health of users and may, therefore, best fall under the purview of the field of public health. New psychoactive drugs reaching the general population have long been a challenge to clinicians and public health officials that are forced to react to an ambiguous problem and relatively unknown substance. While public health officials have successfully addressed historical cases of emerging drugs (see Nicholson and Balster's 2001, concerns about GHB), it seems like the field is constantly behind on prevention and treatment (Spiller et al. 2011). As the time it takes to reformulate a new substance is shorter than the time required for the medicine and health care to study all of the intricacies of its use, public health interventions and medical knowledge will continue to lag behind.

Poison control centers are often the first line of defense made aware of an emerging drug. In recent history, these centers and their associated call lines often report questions about new psychoactive drugs before their clinical effects are well-defined (Vohra et al. 2011). As a result, they are forced to offer advice and guide treatment based on protocols for drugs considered to be similar. This is problematic in that the newer analogues of extant psychoactive substances often have effects on the body that are distinct from similar traditional drugs (Martinez-Clemente et al. 2012; Angoa-Pérez et al. 2012). Furthermore, we must also consider that spikes in calls to poison control centers may be partly a function of unfamiliarity with emerging drugs. For example, if a parent were to catch their child high on marijuana, it is unlikely that he/she would contact a poison control center to obtain medical advice. This should not be a surprise as the parent is likely to have some experience with marijuana (perhaps through their own use or the use of someone they know well). Yet, if this same parent found out their child was high and experiencing wild hallucinations while on Bromo-DragonFly, there is a much greater chance of a phone call to a poison control center or a trip to the emergency room.

In the early stages of a drug's emergence, physicians are equally trailing in preparation and knowledge (Corazza et al.2013). Corazza et al. (2013) suggest that health professionals are consistently at a deficit due to the "absence of up-to-date scientific literature and reliable sources of information." In a recent study of clinicians within fields likely to encounter emerging drug users such as addiction management, emergency medicine, and psychiatry, an overwhelming portion of professionals self-reported a weak or poor understanding of new recreational substances. They were not confident in their ability to identify emerging drug use or dependence (Simonato et al. 2013). For professionals that reported having some knowledge on the subject, the majority of this group reported gathering information from sources that were not peer-reviewed (typically on the Internet).

When medical knowledge about an emerging drug becomes available, it is initially largely based on limited anecdotal information and case studies (Vohra et al. 2011). Users that suffered more severe, untoward, or unique effects are likely overrepresented among these cases. This may obviously lead to biased understandings of the drug and the relevant courses of treatment. Furthermore, the information gathered from cases is likely irrelevant for nontraditional user populations, such as the elderly and very young children. This may force clinicians to assume that the substance is best treated in these populations in the same way as it is for older adolescents and young adults. Laboratory tests for emerging substances may be initially unavailable, inaccurate, or error-prone in early versions, and misinterpreted by undertrained technicians. Additionally, there is a great void of reliable information about dose relationships and potential drug interactions with other recreational drugs, pharmaceuticals, and supplements, particularly in the early stages of emergence.

Even in the best circumstances, clinicians will be forced to make treatment decisions without knowledge of a drug's potency (Vohra et al. 2011). Industrially packaged products may not detail strength, and those that do may describe the product's contents in a nonclinical or inaccurate way. Several studies of recent synthetic emerging drugs have clearly demonstrated that the product's labeling does not always reflect the contents of the package (Dybdal-Hargreaves et al. 2013; Baron et al. 2011; Ayres and Bond 2012). Further, the next generation of emerging drugs may consist of unique chemicals that require reassessment and/or new packaging boasting a new formulation created in an attempt to skirt the law.

Some suggest that the public health burden from emerging drugs may increase after regulation. The transition from licit to banned substance would move marketing from legitimate retail outlets to the black market. As a result, street dealers may increasingly handle these products before it reaches end users; dealers are known to use cutting agents, which may include toxic substances. The increase in impurities and decrease in the awareness of content is likely to lead to negative consequences for users (Winstock et al. 2010). However, those regulating emerging drugs hope to see a net decrease in drug harm due to fewer users through restricting access.

One of the best strategies to manage and combat emerging drug issues may be to utilize the same mediums that are helping to facilitate spread of information promoting the drug. The use of online resources and social media may help to get emerging drug health-related information to potential users. They may also help to convey information to health care professionals who may not otherwise take the time to read scientific information about less frequently used emerging drugs. One of the goals of Recreational Drugs European Network (ReDNet) is to use information and communication technologies to reach health professionals with the latest useful information about novel psychoactive drugs (Corazza et al. 2013). Though its success cannot be fully assessed at this time, ReDNet may become the model for dispersing emerging drug information.

At a time when pharmaceutical and health care supply costs are increasing and the economy is struggling, health care providers are being forced to increase efficiency. Budget cuts and the burden of an aging and obese population have resources stretched thin. This makes adequate preparations for new challenges with new costs difficult, if not impossible. Research and resources are rarely directed at a new problem until it is firmly entrenched as a significant societal concern. As such, the public health and health care reaction to emerging drugs may lag even further behind than necessary. Though the field may improve its ability to manage reactions to some drugs over time, it is important to note that we are still improving our ability to handle drugs that have been around for decades or even centuries. At best, the public health field will improve its reaction time to emerging drugs, but as new products will continue to be formulated, it will never completely catch up (Spiller et al. 2011).

1.6   Divergence from Federal Guidance and Law

In the modern era of drug regulation, and for the vast majority of the last century, US drug control policy was organized and dictated from the federal level. Though the Control Substances Act of 1970 confirmed federal oversight of drug regulation and led to the implementation of our present system, the supervision of drug products truly began in 1906 when the Pure Food and Drug Act regulated product labeling. Since that time, the Federal government has largely taken the lead in initiating law and policy with states following its example. For the most part, this also has been true for emerging substances and drugs just beginning to reach the market. Furthermore, in comparison to the United Kingdom, Australia, and other comparable countries, the US Federal government has historically been among the first to act when new psychoactive drugs emerged (Coulson and Caulkins 2012). Although some attribute this fact to the USA having a better ability to identify and react to emerging problems, it may be the case that use of these drugs first became common in the States or that American culture was more likely to foster a drug scare or moral panic.

The predominant pattern has changed somewhat in the last decade. Most significantly, many contemporary emerging drugs are being addressed internationally before appreciably reaching the USA. Their changes offer some guidance to US decision makers in advance. Yet, this advantage may have fragmented the American response to emerging drugs. Whereas the states once followed the Federal government's lead, it has recently failed to make concrete decisions about emerging drugs. The Drug Enforcement Administration (DEA) has labeled some substances such as salvia and kratom as "drugs of concern," but has offered states little guidance in managing issues related to those chemicals. Even in the cases of emerging drugs eventually banned at the federal level such as synthetic cannabinoids and bath salts, states were the first to act on the issue. This presents an interesting change in drug regulation and may offer insight into how our system of government will address drug issues in the future. In addition to a detailed exploration of the legal and law enforcement issues linked to emerging drugs, Chap. 5 contains a detailed account of this potential systematic change as related to both emerging and traditional street drugs and offers insight into the future form of US drug policy.

1.7 Setting the Tone

Following a comprehensive review and analysis, we present our suggestions for best dealing with the emerging drugs of today. We clearly and concisely offer recommendations for managing emerging drug issues based on historical experiences and discerning deliberation. We also provide our expectations for the future and indicate areas that may need to be focal points for law enforcement, educators, and policymakers. In all, we suggest a proactive approach in monitoring and studying emerging drugs, but a cautious and federal level approach in regulating them.

The advantage in our approach lies in our multidisciplinary background; the following pages dive deep into the problems facing public health, emergency medicine, law enforcement, crime laboratories, drug courts, treatment providers, parents, and recreational drug users. It also uniquely examines how emerging drugs impact the spectrum of players involved in recreational drug use from varying points of view. Through this method, we begin to establish an evidence base to best deal with these issues and hope to spark a well-informed dialog on how to mitigate problems using a multifaceted approach instead of a common reliance on enforcement. We contend that emerging drug threats have unique features that demand a different approach from "traditional" illicit drugs or commonly abused prescription drugs. Importantly, the key players are beginning to acknowledge the dearth of information that exists on this subject. The following begins to address this gap.

References

Angoa-Pérez, M., Kane, M. J., Francescutti, D. M., Sykes, K. E., Shah, M. M., Mohammed, A. M., Kuhn, D. M., et al. (2012). Mephedrone, an abused psychoactive component of 'bath salts' and methamphetamine congener, does not cause neurotoxicity to dopamine nerve endings of the striatum. *Journal of Neurochemistry, 120*(6), 1097–1107.

Arunotayanun, W., & Gibbons, S. (2012). Natural product 'legal highs'. *Natural Product Reports, 29*(11), 1304–1316.

Ayres, T. C., & Bond, J. W. (2012). A chemical analysis examining the pharmacology of novel psychoactive substances freely available over the internet and their impact on public (ill) health. Legal highs or illegal highs? *BMJ open, 2*(4).

Baron, M., Elie, M., & Elie, L. (2011). An analysis of legal highs-do they contain what it says on the tin? *Drug Testing and Analysis, 3*(9), 576–581.

Brandt, S. D., Sumnall, H. R., Measham, F., & Cole, J. (2010). Analyses of second-generation 'legal highs' in the U.K.: Initial findings. *Drug Testing and Analysis, 2*(8), 377–382.

Cone, E. J. (2006). Ephemeral profiles of prescription drug and formulation tampering: evolving pseudoscience on the Internet. *Drug and Alcohol Dependence, 83,* 31–39.

Corazza, O., Demetrovics, Z., van den Brink, W., & Schifano, F. (2012). Legal highs' an inappropriate term for 'Novel Psychoactive Drugs' in drug prevention and scientific debate. *International Journal of Drug Policy, 24,* 82–83.

Corazza, O., Assi, S., Simonato, P., Corkery, J., Bersani, S., Demetrovics, Z., Schifano, F., et al. (2013). Promoting innovation and excellence to face the rapid diffusion of Novel Psychoactive Substances in the EU: The outcomes of the ReDNet project. *Human Psychopharmacology: Clinical and Experimental, 28*(4), 317–323.

Coulson, C., & Caulkins, J. P. (2012). Scheduling of newly emerging drugs: A critical review of decisions over 40 years. *Addiction, 107*(4), 766–773.

Dargan, P. I., Albert, S. & Wood, D.M. (2010). Mephedrone use and associated adverse effects in school and college/university students before the U.K. legislation change. *QJM, 103,* 875–879.

Davies, S., Wood, D. M., Smith, G., Button, J., Ramsey, J., Archer, R., Dargan, P. I., et al. (2010). Purchasing 'legal highs' on the Internet-is there consistency in what you get? *QJM, 103*(7), 489–493.

Detrick, B. (2010). Salvia Takes a Starring Role. *The New York Times.* http://www.nytimes.com/2010/12/26/fashion/26noticed.html. Accessed 27 Nov 2013.

Dillon, N. (2012). Demi Moore 911 call reveals actress was 'semi-conscious' and 'convulsing' after smoking unknown substance. *The Daily News.* http://www.nydailynews.com/entertainment/gossip/demi-moore-911-call-reveals-actress-semi-conscious-convulsing-smoking-unknown-substance-article-1.1012944#ixzz2ettuJPq2. Accessed 27 Nov 2013.

Dybdal-Hargreaves, N. F., Holder, N. D., Ottoson, P. E., Sweeney, M. D., & Williams, T. (2013). Mephedrone: Public health risk, mechanisms of action, and behavioral effects. *European Journal of Pharmacology, 714,* 32–40.

Evren, C., Bozkurt, M., Yavuz, K. F., Yavuz, N., Ulusoy, S., Alnıak, İ., Memetoğlu, M. E., et al. (2013). Synthetic cannabinoids: Crisis of the decade. *Düşünen Adam: The Journal of Psychiatry and Neurological Sciences, 26*(1), 1–11.

Fass, J. A., Fass, A. D., & Garcia, A. S. (2012). Synthetic cathinones (bath salts): Legal status and patterns of abuse. *The Annals of Pharmacotherapy, 46*(3), 436–41.

Griffin, O. H., III., Miller, B. L., & Khey, D. N. 2008. Legally high? Legal considerations of *Salvia divinorum. Journal of Psychoactive Drugs, 40,* 183–191.

Hiaasen, S., & Green, N. (2012). No bath salts detected: Causeway attacker Rudy Eugene had only pot in his system, medical examiner reports. *Miami Herald.* http://www.miamiherald.com/2012/06/27/2871098/mes-report-eugene-had-no-drugs.html. Accessed 27 Nov 2013.

Jerry, J., Collins, G., & Streem, D. (2012). Synthetic legal intoxicating drugs: The emerging 'incense' and 'bath salt' phenomenon. *Cleveland Clinic Journal of Medicine, 79*(4), 258–264.

Johnston, L. D., O'Malley, P. M., Bachman, J. G., & Schulenberg, J. E. (2013). *Monitoring the Future national survey results on drug use, 1975–2012. Volume 1: Secondary school students* (p. 604). Ann Arbor: Institute for Social Research, The University of Michigan.

Khey, D. N., Miller, B. L., & Griffin, O. H. (2008). *Salvia divinorum* use among a college student sample. *Journal of Drug Education, 38*(3), 297–306.

Martínez-Clemente, J., Escubedo, E., Pubill, D., & Camarasa, J. (2012). Interaction of mephedrone with dopamine and serotonin targets in rats. *European Neuropsychopharmacology, 22*(3), 231–236.

Miller, B. L., Boman, J. H., & Stogner, J. (2013). Examining the measurement of novel drug perceptions: *Salvia divinorum*, gender, and peer substance use. *Substance Use & Misuse, 48*(1–2), 65–72.

National Drug Intelligence Center (2011). Synthetic cathinones (bath salts): An emerging domestic threat. Washington, DC. http://www.justice.gov/archive/ndic/pubs44/44571/44571p.pdf. Accessed 27 Nov 2013.

Nicholson, K. L., & Balster, R. L. (2001). GHB: A new and novel drug of abuse. *Drug and Alcohol Dependence, 63*(1), 1–22.

Simonato, P., Corazza, O., Santonastaso, P., Corkery, J., Deluca, P., Davey, Z., Schifano, F., et al. (2013). Novel psychoactive substances as a novel challenge for health professionals: results from an Italian survey. *Human Psychopharmacology: Clinical and Experimental, 28*(4), 324–331.

Singleton, M., Stogner, J., & Miller, J.M. (in press). Awareness of novel drug legality in a young adult population. *American Journal of Criminal Justice.*

Spiller, H. A., Ryan, M. L., Weston, R. G., & Jansen, J. (2011). Clinical experience with and analytical confirmation of "bath salts" and "legal highs" (synthetic cathinones) in the United States. *Clinical Toxicology, 49*(6), 499–505.

Stogner, J. M., & Miller, B. L. (2013). Investigating the 'bath salt' panic: The rarity of synthetic cathinone use among students in the United States. *Drug and Alcohol Review, 32*(5) 545–549.

Sumnall, H. R., Evans-Brown, M., & McVeigh, J. (2011). Social, policy, and public health perspectives on new psychoactive substances. *Drug Testing and Analysis, 3*(7–8), 515–523.

U.S. Food and Drug Administration (FDA) (2013). Q&A on dietary supplements. http://www.fda.gov/Food/DietarySupplements/QADietarySupplements/. Accessed 27 Nov 2013.

Vandrey, R., Stitzer, M. L., Mintzer, M. Z., Huestis, M. A., Murray, J. A., & Lee, D. (2012). The dose effects of short-term dronabinol (oral THC) maintenance in daily cannabis users. *Drug and Alcohol Dependence, 128,* 64–70.

Vardakou, I., Pistos, C., & Spiliopoulou, C. (2011). Drugs for youth via Internet and the example of mephedrone. *Toxicology letters, 201*(3), 191–195.

Vohra, R., Seefeld, A., Cantrell, F. L., & Clark, R. F. (2011). *Salvia divinorum*: Exposures reported to a statewide poison control system over 10 years. *The Journal of Emergency Medicine, 40*(6), 643–650.

Winstock, A., Mitcheson, L., & Marsden, J. (2010). Mephedrone: Still available and twice the price. *Lancet, 376*(9752), 1537.

Chapter 2
Emerging Drugs, Today Versus Yesteryear

Since the 1800s, increasing numbers of new substances have hit the drug scene. Over time, the official responses to these substances have become increasingly more sophisticated. Yet, there still is much to learn from how societies have dealt and continue to deal with the next "scary drug of the year" as there appears to be more similarities than differences in these responses across time and place. While there is a demand for recreational intoxicants in most modern societies, various forces limit the list of legal substances available to those who wish to indulge. The following traces a selection of emerging substances through history to draw attention to the patterns that bridge these cases over time. This exercise will grant us a better focus on our current challenges with the benefit of over a century of hindsight.

2.1 Partitioning Recreational Drugs from Medicine

Delineating the beginnings of *recreational* drug use can be a daunting task. If you were to follow the use of the drugs with the most history— alcohol, marijuana, opium, coca, cocoa, khat, etc.—you would notice that there is a significant entanglement of each drug's central cultural purpose. Many of these substances were used as medicines, in religious ceremonies and sacraments, to enhance social events and, of course, for personal pleasure (Weil 2004). During most times in history, drug use itself was socially acceptable; however, excessive drug use was not. Take, for example, the use of alcohol by ancient Hebrews and early Christians. Wine was central to many ceremonies, family dinners, the Sabbath, and much more. Yet, the problems of abuse and intoxication were woven in the stories of the Old Testament. Even so, most drugs were seen as a gift from God and were treated as such.

As time progressed, there became a clear separation of medicines, *legitimate* recreational products, and prohibited or marginalized drugs for all advanced societies. The reasons for this are varied. For example, Griffin (2012) effectively argues that governments take active steps to protect their citizenry from the potential harm to themselves presented by certain drugs (a "legal paternalism" utilitarian approach) while also protecting others from the harm of drug users/abusers (a "harm to others"

D. N. Khey et al., *Emerging Trends in Drug Use and Distribution*,
SpringerBriefs in Criminology 12, DOI 10.1007/978-3-319-03575-8_2,
© Springer International Publishing Switzerland 2014

utilitarian approach). It is also important to recognize that medical and pharmacological research has become and continues to be a powerful force in defining the
pharmacopeia available to treat physical and mental disease or defect (Courtwright
2009). Generally, these broad forces structure a list of substances that may be used
by physicians to treat their patients or those that are banned from citizen use alto-
gether (among other such forces outside the scope of our argument including racism,
xenophobia, colonization, etc.). Yet, there is still a demand in most societies for
intoxicants for the explicit use of recreation. Alcohol, tobacco, and caffeine products have largely filled that void—creating their own powerful industries—casting
most other psychoactive substances into the margins. When "new" substances hit
the scene, they are quickly relegated to illegality if their main purpose is stereotyped
as *recreational* by the mainstream culture. In fact, there is scant evidence to suggest that even *one* recreational intoxicant has gained mainstream acceptance since
drug laws were put into place. Legislation and rule-making has only favored one
direction: illegality. Marijuana may arguably be a rare exception in certain places;
however, many barriers still exist which prevent marijuana from being accepted as a
product akin to alcohol, tobacco, and caffeine. Even alcohol and tobacco have faced
significant challenges to remain as societies' legitimate intoxicants (e.g., prohibition
and recent public health challenges to tobacco).

Many of the forces shaping this reality in the advanced society have remained
largely unchanged across years of drug discovery and development. The industries
that produce legitimate recreational products for mass consumption have adapted;
being extremely proactive and protective of their fiefdom has ensured their survival.
Many observers take this concept further to claim that the industry is actively com-
plicit with governments to prevent other competing products from emerging (see,
for example, Lee 2012). On the other hand, the medical and pharmaceutical industries have established a firm grip on the pharmacopeia it has developed since the
1800s. Of course, it would not be in their best interest to promote any psychoactive
substance for recreational use. Yet, a perceived fringe element in advanced societies
continues to explore new forms of intoxication. Their motivations for doing so may
have shifted over time, but the outcomes have remained the same: social sanctions,
loss of employment, and/or imprisonment.

The following sections explore the narratives of controversial emerging drugs from
the late 1800s to the 2000s. One theme seems to bridge each narrative—an intoxicant
is identified, its use is perceived to flourish particularly among a seedy element in
society, problems are documented particularly by the media, and a concerted effort
is launched to stamp out its use.

2.1.1 Absinthe

The story of absinthe offers a rich example of the many forces at work that shape
the constructed reality of an emerging psychoactive drug. Absinthe is also one of
the first controversial substances having an excellent historical record for a thorough

postmortem analysis. Yet, this tale begins farther back than many think—as far back as Biblical times. Jad Adams (2004) describes these beginnings vividly: "The righteous are further warned to beware the adulteress, as the writers of Proverbs testify, for though her lips drip honey and her tongue is smoother than oil, ultimately she is more bitter than wormwood and sharp as a two-edged sword." While many ancient medical references cite wormwood—the source for the active psychoactive ingredient thujone in absinthe—as a powerful antiseptic with the added value as an antihelmintic (antiparasitic worm agent), fever reducer, and menstrual pain reliever, there is evidence to suggest that this substance has been mired in controversy for millennia; such a case is supported by folklore and literary references.

By the mid-1600s, drinks containing wormwood were evident in European apothecaries. Yet, wormwood retained a low profile until its explosive use by the French forces in the French Revolution. The conditions of combat in North Africa required French soldiers to spike their water and wine with wormwood extracted into alcohol—a tonic dubbed absinthe by the French. This tonic served as an antimalarial, fought against dysentery, and could be used topically as a natural insecticide. Previously, medical doctors utilized quinine to treat some, not all, of these symptoms; but its true advantage lay in the widespread availability of the plant that produces wormwood in the combat zones. It gave the French Army the edge they needed to succeed, and succeed they did. The intoxicating beverage became tied with victory and patriotism, and this sentiment exploded in France, budding as a major world power.

But it was not *just* intoxication, research points out that the wormwood extract within absinthe added a stimulant-type effect that altered the alcohol effect (for example, see Patočka and Plucar 2003). Yet, legend would have it that users would hallucinate vividly and wildly, a notion captured by artist renditions of "the green fairy" that would become visible while under the influence. To be fair, thujone could potentially cause these behavioral effects at a high dose. However, as Lachenmeier et al. (2008) point out with their chemical analysis of preban absinthes, the thujone levels of popular absinthes in the late 1800s and early 1900s amounted to a mild dose. The key difference was that absinthe was almost always high in alcohol content, typically 150 proof (75 % alcohol). Compared to the other popular alcoholic beverages of the era, absinthe packed the most powerful kick. Those seeking a "high" were certainly in for a good buzz. Think of it this way: one absinthe drink equated to about two to four glasses of wine.

Shortly after the French Revolution, Henri-Louis Pernod made a powerful absinthe widely available as an aperitif. In fact, the company that bears Pernod's name continues to infuse wormwood extract into alcohol using a similar recipe. But this was not always the case; absinthe production came to an abrupt halt in the early 1900s due to a variety of social forces that continue to shape legislation of intoxicating products today, primarily: user base dynamics, industry, governmental agents, the media, and social agents.

Pernod masterfully marketed his absinthe, beginning in 1805, riding the postwar sentiment as if the tonic was a spoil of war. The aperitif originally entered the bourgeoisie and military liquor cabinets, which offered an attractive market to absinthe producers. Note that this initial user base consisted of the affluent, respectable, and sophisticated. By the mid-century mark, many producers had caught on: 25 distilleries were churning out near ten million bottles a year, and each of these producers was advantageously staged for the absinthe craze to come. The French economy was souring, the middle class felt emboldened, and spending cash became increasingly available among the populous. The cafés in Paris blossomed while absinthe became a centerpiece across different factions of the social fabric: military officers, intellectuals, artists, poets, bohemians, and the avant-garde.

This social scene and growing popularity of absinthe became central to its controversy and subsequent ban. Over the years, the drink became less associated with the respectable and more popular with eccentrics, the rebellious, and the marginalized. The most noticeable of the lot were cultural savants, yet social misfits: Verlaine, Rimbaud, Van Gogh, Toulouse-Lautrec, and Gauguin. Gérald de Nerval is a perfect case in point. Nerval was a writer and poet in the early 1800s, who was a part of the growing renaissance for Paris artists and an unforgettable part of the social scene: "Nerval, bizarre to the point of madness, [was] remembered more for walking his pet lobster around the Palais Royale on a blue ribbon than for his verse" (Adams 2004, p. 32). Absinthe became everyone's drink—even "adventurous" women indulged. The vast majority of these young ladies were not prostitutes, but their reputations had tones of ill repute. Who else would be hitting the cafés of Paris getting intoxicated with the bohemians and eccentrics?

The stereotypes associated with the Moulin Rouge in Montmartre, France, began to be associated with absinthe excess. Sexual debauchery, intoxication, irresponsibility, gluttony, and other such sinful indulgencies at the infamous cabaret were fueled by absinthe. As a recent comparison, the Moulin Rouge scene of the 1890s with absinthe resembles the New York dance club Studio 54 in the 1970s with cocaine. The sophisticated aperitif began to fall from grace and became the party monster's favorite vice. At the same time, alcohol sales were flourishing across the country. Adams reports that by 1909, there was an alcohol retail store for every 30 men in the country. Furthermore, almost this entire boom was due to absinthe—use of absinthe had more than doubled since 1885, while the use of all other liquors remained flat (5 % growth during the years 1885 and 1892). Use of absinthe continued to grow among those who could not afford it years earlier. Even the poor and destitute could buy into this trend; liquor producers began to cater to both ends of the consumer spectrum. For the rich, respectable companies, such as Pernod, continued to refine their recipes and offer absinthe created by distilling fine wines and then adding a wormwood preparation. To reach the working class and poor, however, various distillers created products that infused wormwood in low-grade distilled alcohol. Furthermore, these low-grade products were suspected to contain toxic levels of impurities, metals, and poisonous compounds.

Lachenmeier and his colleagues failed to analyze these bottles of bottom-shelf absinthes. Perhaps, these swill brands contained toxins and/or high thujone levels, enabling users to hallucinate but to the detriment of their health. Even if this was not the case, what is important was the growing *perception* that absinthe was causing serious health and societal problems among the populous in the early twentieth century. This was evidenced by a new diagnosis, "absinthism," which was investigated as a syndrome distinct from alcoholism; the drink purported to cause insanity, moral failings, criminality, and sterilization. Essentially, the anti-absinthe movement became a strong part of temperance in France. Wine (which was not as tied with excess) seemed socially acceptable, but absinthe use crossed the line.

The wine industry, reeling from years of loss from a recent widespread fungal epidemic that decimated French vineyards, was finally seeing resurgence in the early twentieth century. It appears that this industry was quietly reveling in the absinthe controversy as their market share began to favor their pockets; perhaps they even carefully stoked the anti-absinthe flames to gain an edge on the market. Thujone soon received regulators' attention, and it took most of the ire of the temperance movement in France. Instead of choosing to regulate potent potables, France chose to limit thujone content to absolute minimal levels. Most premier producers refined their recipes without wormwood, such as Pernod's pastis (an "herbal" liqueur like Jägermeister, Chartreuse, and Anís).

As an emerging drug, absinthe gained a bad reputation when it became associated with the underclass and social deviants. It also symbolized a point in time in which alcohol was being consumed in larger quantities, and more importantly, in a social context that was quite nontraditional (e.g., the spanning cafes on the Boulevard versus the family and/or at religious events). While absinthe hit the mainstream, its popularity did not last. The popularity crested at a time when many nation-states were beginning to become cognizant of substance use and abuse as a societal problem that demanded domestic and international policy development. At this time, governmental regulatory infrastructures were still in their infancy, not extending beyond industries such as banking, finance, and trade. At this key moment in history, problematic drugs (marijuana, opium, cocaine, etc.), including absinthe, were becoming partitioned from legitimate recreational products, and nations were responding by developing ways to manage these problematic substances. As time marched on, the character of absinthe the wonder medical tonic disappeared, to be replaced by absinthe the powerful liquor with an extra devilish psychoactive kick.

Absinthe fits the emerging drug moniker in that (1) it was a "new" substance that truly had unique psychoactive properties different from alcohol and wormwood alone (e.g., old drugs used in a new way), (2) the manner in which an absinthe serving was prepared was entirely new and unique (e.g., pouring absinthe from the bottle into a glass, placing an "absinthe spoon" on top of the glass with a sugar cube, and allowing cool water to drip over the sugar to sweeten the bitterness of the drink while releasing the essential oils from the alcohol into the water—giving the drink its unique cloudy green color), and (3) its use was distinctly recreational in the manner the culture had come to use absinthe. One has to wonder, if governments already had a system in place to identify and regulate dangerous substances, would manufacturers have been allowed to produce and sell absinthe? If so, would it have lasted as a legal recreational product? Absinthe effectively helped to set a precedent on how governments would handle emerging drugs into the twentieth and twenty-first centuries.

It most assuredly would not have been banned if the drink remained in the liquor cabinets of the rich and affluent. Yet, even if that was the case, absinthe's reputation was still suspect in markets outside of France. This was evident by the English perspective on the drink—Adams notes that it became quickly associated with French debauchery, uncouthness, and excess. As such, the English never accepted absinthe as anything but trouble. While absinthe producers expanded its markets into Europe and the USA, it did not appear to reach mainstream status in any other country. Yet, bans spread like wildfire in the early twentieth century as temperance supporters found an easy target in absinthe.

2.1.2 LSD

Of the "new" drugs to surface in the twentieth century, lysergic acid diethylamine (LSD) offers a provocative narrative; the discovery of the drug is well-documented, medical science established a knowledge-base on LSD's potential as a medicine or adjunct to therapy, yet, controversy set in that jeopardized LSD's legitimacy, particularly, as a recreational intoxicant. Soon thereafter, the forces that typically shape drug policy went to work, effectively banning LSD from lawful use.

The tale begins with the work of Dr. Albert Hofmann. While many sources would suggest that Dr. Hofmann discovered the potent hallucinogenic powers of LSD by happenstance on April 16, 1943, Hofmann describes a different story (Hofmann 1970). The clarification he makes in an edited volume in 1970 (and later in a book published in 1980 called "LSD: My problem child") is important; it reflects a need to manage the image of an emerging psychoactive substance:

> "It is often stated in the literature that LSD was discovered by chance. The following account will show that LSD was not the fruit of a chance discovery, but the outcome of a more complex process that had its beginnings in a definite concept, and was followed up by appropriate experiments, during the course of which a chance observation served to trigger off a planned investigation, which then led to the actual discovery. Such a train of events often underlies what is said to be a chance discovery." (Hofmann 1970)

Guided by the principles of scientific inquiry, Hofmann diligently noted the properties of LSD from firsthand experiences. LSD is one of the first hallucinogens created in a laboratory setting and certainly remains the most potent. In retrospect, Hofmann described his experiences under the influence of LSD as a true mystical and spiritual escape from the material world (1993). While he may not have been able to characterize this powerful shift in consciousness and sensation completely when he accidently dosed himself with LSD in 1943, Hofmann knew that this substance had great potential. After years of development work, Sandoz (the pharmaceutical firm based in Switzerland who employed Hofmann) offered free or low-cost samples to scientists with hopes in uncovering clinical applications of what could potentially be a breakthrough substance in mental illness, among other maladies. What occurred over the next two decades is quite remarkable.

Steven Novak (1997) does an excellent job unpacking the complexities in the LSD narrative in the 1950s and 1960s in the USA. According to Novak's thorough research, Dr. Sidney Cohen served as a leading figure in defining LSD's role as a medicine domestically during an era of lax regulations on exploratory drugs. Cohen, a physician with a strong background in pharmacology, came across early LSD research while working at the UCLA School of Medicine. Most of this research detailed the strides investigators were making in using LSD to induce what was perceived to be a "model psychosis" to mimic mental illnesses (and LSD began to be known as a "psychomimetic" agent). Novak notes that these experiences described in the literature did not align with the observations Cohen noted after detailing his firsthand experimentation with LSD. This disconnect led Cohen to tap his social network in search of a resolution; instead of relying on his medically trained colleagues, Cohen reached out to intellectuals (for their gift of self-reflection and prose). This led him to consult with the likes of Aldous Huxley, the famous author who wrote *Brave New World*.

This partnership soon became undermined by personal agendas that grew into conflict. On one side of the spectrum, Cohen tried to procure treatment protocols grounded in science. The "psychomimetic" properties described by earlier researchers were rechristened "psychedelic," a term coined by Huxley in consultation with his friend Humphry Osmond (a Canadian psychologist), meaning "mind-manifesting." These psychedelic experiences were making headway in the late 1950s in psychotherapy, alcoholism treatment, and for the purpose of inspiring creativity in "patients." Novak describes LSD as reaching the peak of medical acceptance in 1959. Yet, in the same time frame, Huxley and the intellectuals were utilizing their connections in the research field to fuel recreational LSD sessions at their homes. Further, pseudoscience "experts" employing LSD "treatment" for various purposes were beginning to flourish in the USA and Canada. Recall that LSD was given for free or at low-cost to legitimate researchers to explore the substance's clinical applications; this was now being exploited for financial gain. Underground laboratories were reported to have been developing LSD illegally (seemingly for the main purpose of recreational use). It seemed like things were getting out of control:

> " ...Cohen did feel 'uncomfortably unscientific.' In 1960 he wrote his sponsor, 'I deplore some of the fringy goings on with this group of drugs.' By then he had distanced himself from some of his associates." (Novak 1997, p. 100)

At about this time, the media began to publish articles and feature television segments on the panacea of LSD "treatment," and this publicity entailed a healthy dose of dramatic embellishments. The combination of these two forces—popularization of LSD by nonmedical zealots and perceived pseudoscientists and the framing of LSD by the popular media as a wonder drug before medical science had adequately vetted it—provided the base for a medical science backlash that led to subsequent controls. Novak notes that this call for action occurred well before the "hippie" counterculture movement, predating Timothy Leary's call to "turn on, tune in, and drop out" and the peak of recreational use.

Sidney Cohen was at the forefront of questioning the safety profile of LSD, at least while under the guidance of conventional medical supervision. In 1960, Cohen published the results of a questionnaire he sent to practitioners actively evaluating LSD in a clinical setting in a paper entitled, "Lysergic acid diethylamide: Side effects and complications." Overall, this research detailed that LSD appeared relatively safe, particularly, when concerning death and suicide (especially suicide—this article was cited by many proponents as a definitive source for LSD's safety profile). Much to Cohen's dismay, many LSD zealots utilized this research to press on with their own (mostly nonmedical) agendas. This point in time demarcated a fork in the road for medical science investigating a potential medicine and lay-LSD enthusiasts (e.g., philosophical and spiritual thinkers as well as common recreational users), many of whom were seeking the mystical forays into the spiritual realm as detailed by influential intellectuals such as Aldous Huxley.

The social context in which LSD was consumed from this moment through the rest of the 1960s progressively got more "fringy," as Dr. Cohen calls it. In the spotlight of this fringe element were two Harvard psychology professors that went rogue, Drs. Richard Alpert and Timothy Leary (Weil 1963). Both professors had become fascinated by the mystic enlightenment that hallucinogens offered, LSD being one key agent in their toolbox. As the undergraduates' curiosity of hallucinogens grew, particularly, given the rumors of Alpert and Leary's experiments with these agents, administrators at Harvard grew nervous. They tried to reign in the professors' efforts, but in the end, felt compelled to fire them both. Alpert and Leary were mired in controversy in that their "experiments" were more like parties while their behavior (particularly, Leary's) became more erratic into the mid-1960s. They established a commune where they based their effort to spread their gospel of using these agents to gain mystic-like enlightenment; the living arrangement itself was strange, let alone the rumored activities that happened on premises.

Enter all of the stereotypes of the counterculture and one can easily see why the mainstream became increasingly concerned about these behaviors and the psychoactive agents that became almost definitive of a "hippie." The counterculture movement that arguably peaked from the "Summer of Love" in Haight-Ashbury (1967) through the end of the decade continued to drive the separation between medical science and nonmedical, drug-fueled alterations of our consciousness to transcend reality, achieving true enlightenment and life-changing epiphanies. Federal regulation attempted to tighten controls on LSD before street popularity began to blossom; however, by that time, LSD had a developing black market manufacturing and distribution system that continued to grow with the counterculture movement. Media publicity performed a complete turnabout from its reports just a few years before. For example, Life magazine ran a cover story entitled, "LSD: The exploding threat of the mind drug that got out of control." Sex, love, and rock'n'roll, drug-induced excess, dismissal of responsible behavior, civil disobedience, etc., none of these things connected with mainstream culture. In fact these social movements challenged the mainstream and the status quo—some would argue somewhat effectively to yield positive social changes. Similar experiences were occurring in Canada, the UK, and Australia, but nothing close to the scope of what was happening in America.

Direct legislative action was taken at the state level (e.g., California in 1966) and federal level (e.g., the Staggers-Dodd amendment to the Food, Drug, and Cosmetics Act in 1968) in order to enhance law enforcement efforts to stamp out nonsanctioned, nonmedical use. From that point on, most medical and pharmaceutical researchers had distanced themselves substantially from LSD and its sister hallucinogenic agents. Just like with absinthe, medicine had moved on to less "risky" substances leaving LSD to fester in its controversy; this move made the hallucinogen an easy target for a legislative ban. In a post-ban era, the use of LSD has remained consistently sporadic in the USA and abroad. That is, a small, but significant subset of adolescents and young adults (primarily) experimented with the substance, but few used LSD often. Even with all of the ire LSD received in the 1960s and the 1970s, it was never a substance that was used substantially relative to other substances, as reported by various national surveys of drug use, nor was it frequently used habitually.

Across various narratives of LSD one can find when investigating the story behind the substance and its eventual ban, one thing remains clear: The manner in which a substance is defined and the primary group responsible for this definition is a key factor in determining a substance's legitimacy. The key to the story is a drug's reputation: from "psychomimetic," psychosis imitation to "psychedelic," mind-manifesting, the applications became central to a substance's identity. From the moment fringe elements crept in, the reputation of LSD became marred, something it has yet to recover from. Thus, the acceptability of an emerging "product" is directly tied to how it comes to market, who uses it, and how they use it. Even if a product is born of science, used in a medical and mainstream manner, and is initially lauded as a "good" drug, a nation can quickly change its mind and ostracize a substance given the right circumstances. The following section explores this very phenomenon.

2.1.3 Quaalude

The perceived boom for drugs in the 1960s was punctuated by the most expansive approach to drug regulation in American history, the Comprehensive Drug Abuse Prevention and Control Act of 1970 (more on this in Chap. 5). As irony would have it, the 1970s would prove to be the decade of excess and widespread use. Many youths and young adults experimented with a widening array of substances for recreational purposes. One of these drugs was an accepted medicine with a brand name of Quaalude (generic name methaqualone). Methaqualone was a potent barbiturate-analogue used primarily to treat insomnia, but it became a problem drug when its popularity increased among recreational drug users.

To begin, barbiturates are a blunt pharmacological tool to reduce anxiety, induce sleep, and treat seizure disorders; in other words, while this class of drugs has medical value, their side effects have kept drug developers hard at work in search of more refined medicines that effectively targeted these individual symptoms without extensive side effects. Methaqualone was intended to offer that solution. It seemed to give physicians a terrific treatment option for anxiety and insomnia, and as an added bonus, it was not technically a barbiturate. It quickly became the drug of choice for the treatment of these symptoms in both the USA and the UK (over a decade of its availability on the market)—it was *the* "safer" alternative to barbiturates. In actuality, however, methaqualone retained a similar safety profile to its chemical cousins in the barbiturate family.

Unlike LSD described above (which posed more of a social threat than a true public health concern), methaqualone posed a significant public health threat—both in terms of clinical and recreational use. The worst aspect of barbiturates and methaqualone was their ability to cause severe physical dependence. Those who abused alcohol and barbiturates together were particularly at risk for overdosing and were subject to severe withdrawal symptoms including death.

Inciardi (1992) argues that recreational users were drawn to the drug because of its overstated safety claims. While the safety claims may be a part of the reason why recreational users increasingly favored methaqualone, it seems more likely that these claims had a more important effect on physicians and regulators. Physicians overprescribed the drug to their patients which exposed countless patients to its euphoric effects and made it readily available to recreational users. Throughout the 1970s, methaqualone became very popular in discothèques and dance clubs in the USA and the UK, making it a commonly used recreational drug. One report (Johnston et al. 1998) estimated that by 1981, about 7 out of 100 college students and 8 out of 100 high school seniors have used methaqualone at least once in the previous year. Many social scenes in which methaqualone was popularly used also featured alcohol consumption. This became a particularly dangerous combination.

Regulation may have caught this sooner; however, regulators chose not to monitor methaqualone closely—that is, until problems surfaced. Even when these problems became trumpeted by the media and made national headlines, regulators were slow to react. Many blame the influence of the pharmaceutical industry, while others cite the lack of sufficient regulatory safeguards to prevent such a public health problem. Either way, recreational use of methaqualone blossomed into the 1970s despite widespread knowledge of its potential harms. Scholars (see Kempton and Kempton 1973; Inciardi 1992; Ray 1978) argue that regulators and the medical community did not heed the available abuse potential of methaqualone. These postmortem evaluations often cite the previous problems exhibited in Japan, Germany, and other countries, yet do not give an accurate understanding of the process of regulatory decision making available at the time. Like with LSD, methaqualone was born of science. While LSD was primarily isolated due to its reputation, methaqualone had an additional problem of being an overall poor pharmacological tool in the pharmacopeia toolkit. It did not target the symptoms it was designed to treat without moderate-to-severe drawbacks. Innovations in sleep and anxiety disorder treatment assured methaqualone's ultimate demise. This also explains why methaqualone is available in other countries, but remains an unpopular choice among prescribing physicians.

Yet, methaqualone became a darling among recreational drug users in the dance scene. It emerged as a harmful drug in this setting and for many years afterwards was routinely used and abused despite its then-known harms. This narrative has become a case study for future medical products whose properties may be what recreational drug users crave (like OxyContin and Xanax, for example). Methaqualone is an example of why the pharmaceutical industry must not only vet products for use as intended, but also must evaluate their potential for misuse and abuse by patients and recreational drug users.

2.1.4   MDMA, Ketamine, and GHB

Other contemporary substances have followed similar pathways as both LSD and methaqualone above. It is also interesting to note that none of them followed the absinthe model. That is, there has not since been one emerging recreational intoxicant that has achieved mainstream success only to be subsequently banned. For example, ecstasy (3,4-methylenedioxymethamphetamine, abbreviated MDMA, also known as molly) followed a similar narrative as LSD in the 1970s and 1980s. In fact, Akers (1992) reports that ecstasy filled the void created by LSD restrictions for mental health providers seeking a chemical adjunct to psychotherapy. The similarities do not stop there—MDMA had almost the same "fringy" experience as LSD with the next generation: Rogue practitioners were using MDMA with their patients, the drug-fueled recreational parties, and MDMA was seeping into the club and dance hall scenes. The most high profile incident to spark regulators' concern came from Dallas, Texas where the self-described "ecstasy missionary" named Michael Clegg began openly promoting and selling the substance. The media quickly caught on and described MDMA as the new LSD for the 1980s with the potential to be the next major drug problem for the USA. Regulators promptly responded by placing MDMA on the banned list of controlled substances (Schedule I) without much regard to its potential medical utility. Similar to LSD, there was not a loud chorus of medical or pharmaceutical support for MDMA during the regulatory hearings on the substance; its fate was largely sealed by crossing the boundary of potential medicine to blatant recreational consumption by nonmainstream factions of society.

Ketamine seems to model methaqualone's emergence pattern, but not completely. Like methaqualone in the 1970s, ketamine became a part of a music scene in the mid-1990s, particularly, in the USA and the UK. However, there are two key differences between the substances' narratives: (1) Ketamine was not as tied to the abuse patterns and, in particular, lethality as methaqualone, and (2) the drug never became nearly as popular—at least, not yet. The Drug Enforcement Administration (DEA) began closely monitoring ketamine's use and abuse patterns in 1995 when the organization listed the substance on its emerging drug list. After 4 years' time, with a noted lack of urgency, regulators decided to list ketamine as a Schedule III substance. This was a far cry from an outright ban. As such, ketamine appears out of line with the other narratives discussed in this text. It should not be surprising, then, to learn that ketamine does have some medical value as a unique anesthetic (Way 1982), particularly, in veterinary medicine (Wright 1982). However, this anesthetic has never been preferred over the various others in our current pharmacopeia. It has remained an option for physicians in both adult and juvenile patient populations, at least for now.

In recent years, public health experts and emergency department physicians have been reporting a rising trend in the untoward effects of ketamine abuse among the recreational population. For example, Chee Kong Ho et al. (2010) published the most recent report on ketamine-induced ulcers and inflammation of the bladder resulting from long-term abuse. This is a report from Malaysia; similar peer-reviewed reports have surfaced from Canada, Belgium, Hong Kong, and Taiwan. To date, these and similar reports have not yet shifted ketamine's scheduling in the USA, Canada, or the UK. The potential for a debate on ketamine to begin in any of these countries is entirely possible; all it needs is a spark. This will begin with a perception of growing nonmedical recreational use, particularly, if the media catches on to its use by marginalized populations, and could end with ketamine being more strongly restricted.

Gamma-hydroxybutyric acid (GHB) is another interesting contemporary case of an emerging drug that caught regulators' attention. This narrative centers on the use of an intoxicating agent to victimize the helpless and vulnerable. In particular, during the late 1980s and in the early 1990s, GHB became known for its use in drug-facilitated sexual assaults becoming classified as a "date rape drug," thus separating it from other recreational drugs at the time. There were two primary contexts for the nonmedical use of GHB during that era: in the club and dance hall scene as a recreational intoxicant and among bodybuilders as a performance-enhancing drug. Similar to methaqualone's narrative, recreational GHB was being used in a context that included alcohol—and, in fact, methaqualone and GHB share similar drug action (e.g., how the chemical affects body systems) and effects, particularly when mixed with alcohol.

There is a key difference with GHB relative to methaqualone, however; like ketamine, US regulators decided to keep an FDA-approved version of GHB (a pill called Xyrem) legal, but controlled, as a Schedule III drug. Thus, these are two rare instances in which the medical and pharmaceutical communities have been able to claim that an emerging substance that has slipped into the recreational domain could be used safely with the supervision of a physician. The liquid form of GHB, purported to be the culprit of date rapes across the country, was completely banned.

This decision may make better sense with some additional context. Other notable "date rape drugs," such as Rohypnol (generic name: flunitrazepam) and other benzodiazepines are scheduled in a similar, or even less scrupulous manner. Furthermore, the abuse patterns of both ketamine and GHB never reached the levels seen with methaqualone. In fact, since regulators have scheduled these drugs, the recreational use of these substances plummeted to near-zero levels. MDMA, on the other hand, remains relatively popular in the twenty-first century despite its Schedule I status. While it would be foolhardy to attribute these differences solely to the regulatory distinctions, particularly since MDMA's effects are perceived as more desirable by users, these cases do reinforce that more strict regulation does not equate to more effective regulation.

2.2 Drug Scares and the Media

Each of these examples above has a common thread. Many scholars have pointed out the similar manner in which the press handles these emerging drugs. For the most part, a particular language and tone bridges all of these cases. Presenting many of these cases as "an epidemic," "outbreak," "scourge," "plight," the press often make dire claims of spreading addiction, misery, and irrational behavior. These messages also accompany ties to crime, violence, and social deviance. In many circumstances, there are truths behind these claims of drug threats; however, the entire picture is rarely offered to viewers/readers. Even policy makers may have a hard time finding sound resources at their fingertips when determining a course of action in handling these perceived threats. In 1992, Akers put this phenomenon succinctly:

> Which of these substances, or others we have not yet heard about, will turn out to become widely used and the focus of law enforcement, education, and treatment programs remains to be seen. As the new threats appear, we need to learn from the past history of the scary drugs of the year. Those lessons are twofold: First, the more hysterical alarms should be greeted with skepticism … We have seen drug scares come and go; epidemics develop, peak, and decline with few of the horrors predicted coming true. Second, the potential dangers of each drug should be taken seriously. Often there is real, substantive basis for the alarm, even though it may get exaggerated or distorted … The assumption that the public perception is always wrong or simply media hype is not warranted. Blasé assurances about harmlessness and safety of drugs by those attempting to debunk the beliefs of a gullible public are also not justified by the history of the scary drug of the year. (pp. 42–43)

Just like with any policy-making, there are pushes and pulls that help shape the process and the end result. Typically, the only thing preventing an outright ban for an emerging substance is some level of existing medical use. It appears that the promise of future medical use is quite insignificant to policymakers relative to the perceived or actualized harms tied to an emerging substance. On the other side of the fulcrum lies the multiplicity of justifications for regulating these substances: physical and/or psychological harm (actualized or perceived), addiction, harm to youths, family disintegration, interpersonal violence, sexual deviance and depravity, and grave bodily injury or death. Thus, it should not be surprising that any substance used recreationally without substantial legitimate use has been fast-tracked for a ban (typically) or heavy restriction (atypically).

For politicians in developed countries, the decision to restrict these substances becomes commonsense. Constituents have not historically railed against restricting emerging drugs. There have been political consequences for those that have taken action on mainstream recreational substances, but even these actions are limited. Take the recent restrictions on tobacco as an example. In 2010, the Food and Drug Administration was successful in bringing about restrictions on the tobacco industry such as prohibiting the sale of packages with fewer than 20 cigarettes, enhancing the restrictions on tobacco vending machines, and curtailing marketing and promotions of tobacco companies. Even in light of major lobbying efforts, the tobacco industry has had a difficult time curtailing restrictions targeting their most youthful clients. It was not long ago that these efforts have fallen flat—the Food and Drug Administration diligently tried to move on curtailing the advertisement and marketing efforts of the tobacco industry (particularly the kinds that target youths and young adults) in 1996. This led to a major settlement in 1998; however, it took over a decade for public health officials and regulatory agencies to further side step the barriers put in place by the industry to pass Regulations Restricting the Sale and Distribution of Cigarettes and Smokeless Tobacco to Protect Children and Adolescents (Federal Register 2010). Without such lobbying ability, imagine how effortless it is to place restrictions on an obscure and unpopular substance.

Taking strides to restrict the latest scary drug of the year seems like an easy decision on the surface level. Almost by rule, however, these decisions are not grounded in empirical evidence. The unintended consequences of these unilateral decisions reside mostly in the expended resources involved in regulating an ever expanding list of controlled substances. In many cases, the media is involved in amplifying the perceived scope of emerging drug use. They also serve as a conduit for anecdotal evidence that often fuels legislative and administrative hearings on emerging drugs. Omitting hype, anecdotal evidence, and hysteria, the following section outlines a typology of emerging drugs. It also assigns a threat level to each given the historical context of each typology.

2.3   Current Trends

At a point when the pharmacopeia of developed nations have reached a point of maturity, emerging drugs can easily be classified into the following broad categories: newly synthesized analogues, rediscovered botanicals, and modified classics. Observers must also keep in mind that regulation regimes have also reached maturity. Thus, agencies such as the DEA have a broad idea of what they are looking for before they act on an up and coming substance that may require action: absence of empirically known medical use and potential harm by the way of physical injury and/or dependence liability. Thus, the highest likelihood of a response to any emerging drug would meet these criteria: (1) receives a particular threshold of attention, (2) is not born of acceptable contemporary medical/pharmaceutical research, and (3) is perceived to have the capability of causing harm.

2.3.1   Newly Synthesized Analogues

The emerging drug phenomenon of the twenty-first century centers on a multifaceted group of substances that can be broadly categorized as *newly synthesized analogues*. Typically, these compounds are slight-to-moderate alterations of existing controlled substances that require a moderate-to-advanced understanding of chemistry to produce. They are also vastly unlikely to be the focus of any serious mainstream medical research, but may have been investigated by pharmaceutical firms at one point. Partly for this reason, these substances have been clandestinely produced with increasing frequency by producers in the Far East (China, India, Pakistan, and Japan, for example). A quick Internet search for code terms, such as "research chemicals," will give someone a glimpse of the variety of substances available for purchase through a foreign agent (at the time of this writing, such websites include drsynthetic.com, brc-finechemicals.com, researchchemicalsonlinestore.com, and researchchemicals.net).

While the code term "research chemicals" largely includes a range of substances that mimic MDMA (ecstasy), MDA (a precursor to and cousin of ecstasy), ketamine, PCP (a cousin of ketamine), and similar known illicit drugs, newly synthesized analogues can include an entire range of hybrids of different distinct drug classes. For example, in the "tryptamine" section of researchchemicals.net, one can find the substance "5-MeO-DALT," which is purported to have a drug action similar to psilocybin mushrooms and DMT (both potent hallucinogens) with distinctive stimulant properties. Many of these substances have been popularized by cult classic books by rogue chemist Alexander Shulgin (see Shulgin and Shulgin 1991, 1997; see also an interview with Shulgin by Morris and Smith 2010). Many underground chemists have emulated his practices (Morris 2011), and for many years, their efforts have been the fodder of Internet forums across the globe without most people noticing—even most drug users. Other chemists, many contributing in the same forums, have focused on analogues of other drugs, like marijuana (synthetic cannabinoids), cocaine, and methamphetamine (synthetic stimulants). At some point, entrepreneurial people who were extremely nonadverse to risk took notice and began to set up production and distribution schemes to take advantage of the void in clear legislation preventing these practices. More discussion on this issue will be presented in the following chapter.

Geographically, much of the production and distribution of these products began outside of the USA. Thus, it should not be surprising that the lion share of newly synthesized analogues has thrived in Europe before many have reached the USA. The cathinone derivatives are a perfect case in point where Europe, the UK in particular, was reacting to domestic problems with these synthetic stimulants (and various other "research chemicals") far in advance of the USA. On the other hand, synthetic cannabinoids seems to have shared a global timeline: This potential threat surfaced around 2008 causing a storm in interest and concern (see Office of National Drug Control Policy 2013). Thus, recent extant literature by American researchers tends to primarily focus on synthetic cannabinoids.

According to a recent Office of National Drug Control Policy (2013) report, the USA identified 158 "new" synthetic substances in 2012: 51 of which are "new" synthetic cannabinoids, 36 were synthetic cathinones, and 76 were other analogues. While many of these substances were not initially synthesized in 2012 and did not come out of nowhere, there is substantial evidence of a broader array of these substances in the marketplace (primarily, the gray and black markets). Of these emerging threats, synthetic cannabinoids has seen the highest and most marked increases in use by American youth: The most recent Monitoring the Future study results show that more than one in ten high school seniors have used synthetic cannabinoids in the past year, roughly equating to all past-year hallucinogen, ecstasy, and cocaine use combined.

Previously marketed under the brand names like "Spice" and "K2," synthetic cannabinoid products consist of a liquid formulation of one or a combination of "cannabinoid receptor agonists," agents that stimulate the same neurochemical pathways in our bodies as marijuana, sprayed on dried plant matter or similar substrate ("Spice" packaging listed such plant ingredients as blue lotus, red clover, and rose, among others). These products quickly established recreational use patterns that could sufficiently support the argument that they were becoming a substitute for marijuana, particularly, when users were blocked access to marijuana for a litany of reasons: workplace drug screens (de Jager et al. 2012), criminal justice surveillance (e.g., probation, parole, drug court, and treatment compliance; see Cary 2010; Perrone et al. 2012; Rodrigues et al. 2013), or similar circumstances (for example, drug testing in both public and private secondary schools).

As a subtype of emerging drugs, the newly synthesized analogues will be the most likely of all to cause governments headaches until successful strategies of their management are established and executed. To use the language of users, "bath salts" and "fake pot" are only the beginning of many more drugs to come down the pike.

2.3.2 New to Us—Botanicals

On the other hand, emerging drug products of a natural origin generally tend to cause less of a stir. Many of these substances have roots in aboriginal healing practices from a variety of old cultures across the globe: khat, *S. divinorum*, kava, betel, ephedra, morning glory, nutmeg, and many more. While most of these natural medicinal products lay dormant, some become emerging drugs when their "rediscovery" crosses a threshold of attention and after being perceived as doing harm or having the potential to do so. Due to their aboriginal roots, potential linkages to Eastern medicine, and/or inclusion in homeopathic or "alternative medicine" regimens, an almost automatic nonscientific and nonmedical (more specifically, nonconventional medicine) stigma becomes attached to these products.

One of these substances, ephedra, was actually marketed in a legitimate manner by a variety of natural health firms until medical research uncovered its connection to heart damage and distress. Many others, that are mildly psychoactive in character, continue to be legitimately marketed today. Yet, a small subset of these natural medicinal products has marked psychoactive properties that make them likely to be favored by recreational users. Only a small handful of these products exist in stores in the USA and in Europe. The popular ones currently include kratom and kava. At first, products like these led the "legal high" phenomenon as evidenced by Internet search results in the early 2000s (see Halpern and Pope 2001; Dennehy et al. 2005). Yet, it seems that newly synthesized analogues will continue to dominate the emerging drug phenomenon into the future.

2.3.3   New Tricks for Old Drugs

Innovation has been a consistent feature of drug use as users have notoriously searched for longer, more efficient, and intense highs. Along with including novel substances in our definition of emerging drugs, we also include traditional substances that are being used in new ways. Two recent examples of this trend have been the nontraditional consumption of alcohol through the use of an inhaler device or suppositories and the new practice of "dabbing" with butane-extracted hash oil. Through new methods of consumption comes a concern over the safety and legality of these practices and the substances in general.

Alcohol accounts for more than 80,000 deaths annually and an estimated US\$ 223.5 billion in damages (CDC 2013), but serves mainly as one of the "legitimate" recreational highs. This status has been preserved largely by the ability of users to moderate their consumption. A recent trend in adolescent alcohol use involves engaging in innovative ways to consume alcohol more efficiently. A practice referred to as "smoking" alcohol has reportedly become popular in recent years, which involves pouring liquor on dry ice and either directly inhaling or using a lid or straw to either inhale through the mouth or nose. This practice is not entirely new. In 2004, alcohol without liquid (AWOL) devices began appearing on the market. Erroneously called "vaporizers," these devices actually act as a nebulizer mixing the alcohol with oxygen into a mist so that it can be inhaled through the lungs. In 2005, Michigan was the first state to ban these devices, and since that time, at least 25 states have banned similar type devices. Inhaling alcohol is especially dangerous because a higher dose of alcohol is sent to the brain bypassing organs responsible for initially metabolizing it (called first-pass metabolism) like the stomach and liver. Additionally, the body loses its primary safety mechanism against alcohol poisoning—vomiting—as the alcohol no longer is absorbed through the gastrointestinal tract.

The original AWOL machines were designed to allow only small amounts of alcohol to be inhaled and over a long duration (20 min). Bar owner Steve Baskinger of the Bask Bar and Grill in Wet Paterson, New Jersey purchased one of these devices for his establishment, but soon returned it arguing it did not provide enough of a kick. Despite the legality and ineffectiveness of these devices, the primary reason for not gaining widespread popularity is likely due to the false advertising of reduced caloric intake and their hefty price tag. New forms of these devices still exist—like the Vaportini—and are able to bypass the regulations for AWOL devices as they use a different mechanism for vaporizing alcohol (and have an attractively low US\$ 35 price tag). The simple device has a glass globe on top of a glass with a candle inside. The candle heats the globe filled with a shot of liquor and then is inhaled through a straw.

Marijuana remains the most widely used "illicit" drug in the USA, and although it would not typically be considered an emerging drug, modern innovations in marijuana use do pose some serious questions as it moves toward legal status. Marijuana as an illicit drug has been challenged in recent years with 19 states and the District of Columbia allowing medical marijuana, 17 states and several localities allowing some form of depenalization of recreational marijuana, and two states moving toward the legalization of recreational use. Marijuana remains a Schedule I substance under the Controlled Substance Act of 1970 (CSA), but as we discuss in more detail in Chap. 5, the Federal government seems to be allowing states to diverge on marijuana policy. The increased acceptance of recreational use in Colorado and Washington along with the large number of medical marijuana states have allowed new innovations in the forms of marijuana products. A large number of new products have become available at medical dispensaries including edible marijuana products such as baked goods, suckers, hard candy, candy bars, sodas, tea, coffee, and breath sprays. Some have criticized these products for containing high quantities of concentrated amounts of tetrahydrocannabinol (THC), and that this may pose new dangers to users. This is particularly an area of concern with the first marijuana retail stores in Colorado opening in 2014.

Even more concerning is a recent trend in marijuana consumption involving the use of butane-extracted hash oil (BHO) sometimes referred to as "budder," "shatter," or "wax," for the texture of the resulting product. BHO is produced by extracting natural cannabinoids using a butane gas solvent creating a concentrated resin that can contain more than 80 % THC. For reference, the typically marijuana sold on the streets contains about 3 %, with higher grades being about 4–8 %, hashish contains about 8–14 %, and conventional hash oil has up to about 50 %. A new practice referred to by users as "dabbing" involves dipping a metal rod into BHO and then heating up the "dab" using either a specialized device known as an "oil rig" or a modified pipe, bong, or vaporizer and inhaling the vapors produced. Inhaling a small amount of BHO (a dab) according to users can produce a high similar to smoking an entire joint. Even very experienced marijuana users compare dabbing to "getting high for the very first time. Your head spins, your eyes get fluttery, a few beads of sweat surface on your forehead and, suddenly, you're *cosmically* baked" (Breathes 2013:1). As an emerging drug, dabbing is a new modification in the method of intake for marijuana similar to innovations in alcohol consumption through vaporizing. These new techniques of administering a recreational drug, typically used in moderation, may challenge their legality and require further regulations. Further, marijuana activists trying to increase the legal availability of marijuana fear that dabbing might hurt their cause with users experiencing more potent effects, devices resembling crack pipes, and amateur chemists in BHO operations experiencing meth-lab like explosions (Breathes 2013).

2.4   Connecting the Past to the Present

The emerging drugs of yesteryear—such as absinthe, LSD, methaqualone, MDMA, ketamine, and GHB—have been unique lessons to decision makers of the potentiality of "regulation deficiencies." That is, in absence of any or sufficient safeguards, both perceived (e.g., socially constructed) and actualized harms evolve, largely resulting in a routinized drug scare that occurs every so many years. Some of these scares should have been taken very seriously while others seemed like decision makers heeding to those crying wolf. Obviously, it is much easier analyzing these patterns postmortem; however, there are lessons here that will assist us in responding in contemporaneous problems as they arise in the future.

First, build an understanding of how these substances are being used by subcultures. Be particularly vigilant of how substances are being combined, if at all. Methaqualone is an example of an emerging substance, that when mixed with alcohol, becomes incredibly problematic and potentially deadly. Second, understand that there has always been a demand for recreational products and alcohol, tobacco, and caffeine do not seem to be satiating these desires. Just because a substance is psychoactive and may not have a medical use does not mean that decision-makers should automatically ban it. LSD and MDMA, for example, are still effectively stigmatized to the point where legitimate medical research on these substances remains incredibly difficult despite recent breakthroughs in treating trauma-induced psychological disorders. Last, and most importantly, there needs to be an understanding of the forces that shape policy-making in order to be able to steer commonsense decisions on emerging drugs in the future.

References

Adams, J. (2004). Hideous absinthe: A history of the devil in a bottle. London: IB Tauris Publishers.

Akers, R. L. (1992). Drugs, alcohol, and society: Social structure, process, and policy. Belmont: Wadsworth Publishing Company.

Breathes, W. (June 20, 2013) Crazy-high times: The rise of hash oil, meet the golden goop that gets you cosmically baked. Rolling Stone. Available at: http://www.rollingstone.com/culture/news/crazy-high-times-the-rise-of-hash-oil-20130610.

Cary, P. (2010). Spice, K2 and the problem of synthetic cannabinoids. *National Drug Court Institute*, *6*(1), 1–2.

Centers for Disease Control and Prevention. (2013b). Alcohol use and health. Retrieved from http://www.cdc.gov/alcohol/fact-sheets/alcohol-use.htm. Accessed 27 Nov 2013.

Courtwright, D. T. (2009). Forces of habit: Drugs and the making of the modern world. Cambridge: Harvard University Press.

de Jager, A. D., Warner, J. V., Henman, M., Ferguson, W., & Hall, A. (2012). LC-MS/MS method for the quantitation of metabolites of eight commonly-used synthetic cannabinoids in human urine-An Australian perspective. *Journal of Chromatography B*, *897*, 22–31.

Dennehy, C. E., Tsourounis, C. & Miller, A. E. (2005). Evaluation of herbal dietary supplements marketed on the internet for recreational use. *Annals of Pharmacotherapy 39*(10), 1634–1639.

Federal Register. (2010). Regulations restricting the sale and distribution of cigarettes and smokeless tobacco to protect children and adolescents. Available at: https://www.federalregister.gov/articles/2010/03/19/2010-6087/regulations-restricting-the-sale-and-distribution-of-cigarettes-and-smokeless-tobacco-to-protect. Accessed 27 Nov 2013.

Griffin, O. H. (2012). Is the government keeping the peace or acting like our parents? rationales for the legal prohibitions of GHB and MDMA. *Journal of Drug Issues*, *42*(3), 247–262.

Halpern, J. H., & Pope, H. G. (2001). Hallucinogens on the Internet: A vast new source of underground drug information. *American Journal of Psychiatry*, *158*(3), 481–483.

Ho, C. C. K., Pezhman, H., Praveen, S., Goh, E. H., Lee, B. C., Zulkifli, M. Z., & Isa, M. R. (2010). Ketamine-associated ulcerative cystitis: A case report and literature review. *The Malaysian Journal of Medical Sciences: MJMS*, *17*(2), 61.

Hofmann, A. (1970). The discovery of LSD and subsequent investigations on naturally occurring hallucinogens. In Ayd, F. J. & Blackwell, B. (Eds.). Discoveries in biological psychiatry. Lippincott. http://www.psychedelic-library.org/hofmann.htm.

Inciardi, J. A. (1992). The war on drugs II: The continuing epic of heroin, cocaine, crack, crime, AIDS, and public policy (Vol. 2). Mountain View: Mayfield Publishing Company.

Johnston, L., O'Malley, P. M., & Bachman, J. G. (1998). National survey results on drug use from the Monitoring the Future Study, 1975–1997 (Vol. 1). National Institute on Drug Abuse, U.S. Department of Health and Human Services, Public Health Service, National Institutes of Health.

Kempton, R. J., & Kempton, T. (1973). Methaqualone abuse: An epidemic for the seventies. *Journal of Drug Education, 3*(4), 403–413.

Lachenmeier, D. W., Nathan-Maister, D., Breaux, T. A., Sohnius, E. M., Schoeberl, K., & Kuballa, T. (2008). Chemical composition of vintage preban absinthe with special reference to thujone, fenchone, pinocamphone, methanol, copper, and antimony concentrations. *Journal of agricultural and food chemistry, 56*(9), 3073–3081.

Lee, M. A. (2012). Smoke signals: A social history of Marijuana-Medical, Recreational and Scientific. USA: Simon and Schuster.

Morris, H. (2011). Interview with a ketamine chemist. Vice Magazine. http://www.vice.com/magazine/18/2. Accessed 27 Nov 2013.

Morris, H., & Smith, A. (2010). The last interview with Alexander Shulgin. Vice Magazine. http://www.vice.com/magazine/17/5. Accessed 27 Nov 2013.

Novak, S. J. (1997). LSD before Leary: Sidney Cohen's critique of 1950s psychedelic drug research. *Isis, 88*, 87–110.

Office of National Drug Control Policy. (2013) Fact sheet: Synthetic drugs. http://www.whitehouse.gov/ondcp/ondcp-fact-sheets/synthetic-drugs-k2-spice-bath-salts.   Accessed   27 Nov 2013.

Patočka, J., & Plucar, B. (2003). Pharmacology and toxicology of absinthe. *Journal of Applied Biomedicine, 1*, 199–205.

Perrone, D., Helgesen, R. D., & Fischer, R. G. (2012). United States drug prohibition and legal highs: How drug testing may lead cannabis users to Spice. *Drugs: education, prevention and policy, 20*(3), 216–224.

Ray, O. (1978). Drugs, Society, and Human Behavior. St. Louis, MO: C. V. Mosby.

Rodrigues, W. C., Catbagan, P., Rana, S., Wang, G., & Moore, C. (2013). Detection of synthetic cannabinoids in oral fluid using ELISA and LC-MS-MS. *Journal of analytical toxicology, 37*(8), 526–533.

Shulgin, A., & Shulgin, A. (1991). PiHKAL: A chemical love story. Berkeley: Transform Press.

Shulgin, A., & Shulgin, A. (1997). *TiHKAL: The continuation.* Berkeley: Transform Press.

Way, W. L. (1982). Ketamine—its pharmacology and therapeutic uses. *Anesthesiology, 56*(2), 119–136.

Weil, A. T. (1963). The strange case of the Harvard drug scandal. *Look, 27*, 38–48.

Weil, A. (2004).The natural mind: A revolutionary approach to the drug problem. USA: Houghton Mifflin Harcourt.

Wright, M. (1982). *Pharmacologic effects of ketamine and its use in veterinary medicine [Anesthesia]. Journal of the American Veterinary Medical Association, 180*, 1462–1471.

Chapter 3
Emerging Drug Trade and Use: Manufacturing, Marketing, and Understanding Novel Highs

One of the more difficult issues facing decision makers in regard to recent emerging drug threats is the novel nature of their manufacturing process, marketing tactics, distribution schemes, and even the large range and diverse nature of the players in each of these arenas. That is, at every stage of traditional drug control and interdiction modifications must be made to be able to monitor these emerging products. The following section describes this new marketplace with the most current intelligence and research and gives some insight into the scope and logic of novel high production, distribution, and use.

3.1 The Shadow Industry Profiting from Emerging Drug Use

There is no doubt that a large, global industry has been firmly established to cash in on emerging drug markets. Just as an example, recent intelligence from an investigation of a large-scale local and Internet distribution operation in Tempe, Arizona found that the Internet sales alone amounted to about US$ 8,000 per day (US Attorney's Office 2013). Joint investigations by federal agencies (such as the Drug Enforcement Administration, Immigration and Customs Enforcement, US Postal Inspection Service, Attorney General's Office, etc.) have indicated that manufacturers of a variety of emerging drugs primarily reside in developing countries or in the Far East (India, China, Pakistan, and others) and almost always have a foreign origin. Also, these substances often have a principle transit country (e.g., another foreign port of entry) before reaching its destination (US Department of Justice 2011). The global drug intelligence community is still putting together the pieces of who is responsible and defining the upper-level organizational structure behind the shadow industry. More is known about domestic suppliers and distributors at this time, including the scope and scale of domestic operations and how much profit is involved.

It is not only psychoactive substances that drive this phenomenon, although it is one of the more lucrative aspects of this emerging marketplace. In fact, this trend is indicative of a broader phenomenon with large public health implications that we are only beginning to grapple with; health foods, dietary supplements, and herbal

D. N. Khey et al., *Emerging Trends in Drug Use and Distribution,*
SpringerBriefs in Criminology 12, DOI 10.1007/978-3-319-03575-8_3,
© Springer International Publishing Switzerland 2014

biomedicines have all cashed in on loopholes and by bending the rules to bring potentially dangerous drugs to market. Americans spend more than US$ 28 billion a year on what are often assumed to be safe and effective supplements (Cohen 2012). These products often make hefty claims about their abilities to reduce weight, build muscle, improve mental abilities, or improve sexual performance. With more than 100 million American consumers taking some form of vitamin, mineral, herbal ingredient, amino acid, or other naturally occurring ingredient, this growing industry has surprisingly remained effectively unregulated. The Dietary Supplement Health and Education Act of 1994 (DSHEA) defines dietary supplements as including "established ingredients" meaning that these ingredients were sold in the USA prior to 1994 and, therefore, can be sold without evidence of their safety or efficacy (Cohen 2012). For new ingredients, the manufacturer must provide the Food and Drug Administration (FDA) with evidence that there is a "reasonable expectation of safety" (Cohen 2012). Yet, this provision has gone grossly unenforced. Since the passage of DSHEA the number of available dietary supplements increased from 4,000 to more than 55,000, but the FDA has only received notification of approximately 170 new supplement ingredients during that time. This raises large questions about how many of the 51,000 new supplements contain novel and inadequately evaluated ingredients (Cohen 2012). In 2011, the FDA took some steps to try to clarify the level of evidence required to assess safety for novel substances including treating synthetically produced replica of existing compounds as a new ingredients; many still believe the FDA is not doing enough to regulate these products (Cohen 2012).

Take, for example, Zoltrex, a sexual enhancement supplement containing *Ophioglossum polyphllous* as indicated on its label. This product was sold under brand names like Stiff Nights and OMG, with claims like: "Stiff Nights is an all-natural male enhancement supplement that does not require a prescription and may help to increase a man's sexual performance with his partner" (Stiff Nights 2013). After some time on the market, an independent analysis surfaced which indicated that this supplement did not include even trace amounts of ophioglossum (adder's tongue). Ophioglossum had been approved as a dietary ingredient, but Zoltrex's active ingredient consisted of sulfoaildenafil instead. This substance is an analogue of sildenafil (the active ingredient in Viagra), which actually has never gone through FDA testing on humans to this date. Thousands of individuals (as a conservative estimate) may have consumed "Stiff Nights" product prior to its recall (Cohen 2012).

Instead of lying about what a product actually contains, many in the shadow industry have attempted to bypass FDA regulations by marketing a product as "not for human consumption." Importantly, shadow industry firms are still able to get the message to their potential customers of the products' actual intent. New supplements, vitamins, or diet aids may be marketed in this way to avoid the expenses and time delays associated with development, quality assurance, quality control, and, most especially, meeting safety regulations. Manufacturers may even boast that their labeling is linked to better service and pricing: "Because . . . botanical herbal incense is not technically classified as a food or a drug . . . [we] can offer products to the market directly at an affordable price" (The North American Herbal Incense Trade Association 2013). However, it is also a loophole used to get psychoactive products to consumers. Since analogues of banned substances are only technically illegal in the USA if they are explicitly banned or marketed for human consumption, they remain quasi-legal if they are chemically distinct and advertised as having an alternative purpose. In many cases, the alternative advertised use is never truly intended as an actual use and instead is a thinly veiled attempt to circumvent regulation. This is the reason that cathinones were initially labeled "bath salts," many cannabinoids have been advertised as incense or potpourri, and research chemicals are sold for "analytical purposes" or for "in vitro research."

Whether the products reaching consumers in this way are psychoactive or not, they may endanger both users and nonusers. The news media and political players are rightfully most concerned with psychoactive substances since their use may result in direct and immediate health harms, violence, or impaired vehicular operation. But the potential detriment of unregulated health products extends beyond wasted money. Widespread use of unevaluated health supplements may lead to injury, illness, unexpected drug interactions, increased medical noncompliance (patients using novel products as replacements for prescribed legitimate medicine), vehicular accidents, increased health system costs, and an array of other problems. Though these products are somewhat external to the scope of this text, academics and policymakers should be aware that manufacturers of nonpsychoactive substances often take advantages of the same policy inadequacies as those marketing psychoactive ones and that any alteration to policy will affect both.

A shadow industry clearly exists in what may be described as a legal gray area. While manufacturers and dealers largely conform to the letter of the law, they denigrate its intent. The motive of profit reins over health concerns and public interests. As long as the production of "legal highs" and unregulated health supplements remains profitable, we will likely continue to see new psychoactive substances reaching consumers and potentially dangerous supplements filling more and more retail shelf space. The following sections detail how the shadow industry often stays one step ahead of the law, how products are manufactured, and how they reach consumers.

3.1.1 Drug Development and the Regulate and Reformulate Game

There is a dearth of information about how newly synthesized analogues and modified botanicals are researched and evaluated by their producers. This is not surprising given that designers and manufacturers operate on the fringes of the law and production most frequently occurs in developing countries. In many cases, the psychoactive product they market may simply be a compound that, using the language of Wiley et al. (2011), they "hijacked" from legitimate science. Synthetic cannabinoids and many other substances recently marketed as "legal highs" were first created as part of well-intended research studies (Parker et al. 1998; Wiley et al. 2011). Academic reports of those substances' inherent psychoactivity may have helped facilitate their transition to recreational use. Individuals willing to engage in the production of recreational drugs likely accessed academic studies prior to recreating the compounds or creating an analogue. Other compounds may be designed by shadow industry researchers trying to create analogues of natural psychoactive compounds or tweaking extant psychoactive synthetics. Yet another (and more plausible) alternative, sophisticated enthusiasts such as Alexander Shulgin promulgate hundreds of psychoactive compounds complete with a description of their properties, psychoactive effects, side effects, and, as with Shulgin's work, a rating scale of psychoactivity and pleasurability (from personal experimentation with *all* of these substances). Just like how "The Anarchist Cookbook" and "Steal This Book" connected with anti-government types, "PiHKAL" (Phenethylamines i Have Known and Loved, published in 1991) and "TiHKAL" (Tryptamines i Have Known and Loved, published in 1997) connects with rogue underground chemists. Over the years, these efforts have become commercialized by a shadow industry that is reaping the benefits of providing psychoactive substances to customers while skirting the laws restricting this practice. Shulgin's work, among others, provides an elaborate instruction manual to anyone with moderate chemistry skills, some business sense, and little aversion to risk to get started in the shadow industry.

One of the biggest concerns among those in the medical community is that the drugs developed by the shadow industry do not undergo the same rigorous tests as pharmaceutical products but, due to their packaging and availability in stores, are perceived by consumers to be safe regulated products. Neither websites promoting specific products nor packaging materials typically offer any empirical support of their claims (Ginsburg et al. 2012). Even if evidence was provided, its veracity often could not be ascertained due to production and testing likely occurring in developing countries. As such, it is impossible to know whether products underwent any extended testing or trials. There can be no assurances of safety or that the products will not negatively interact with other drugs or medications.

Assuming that the substance manufactured during initial production runs only carried minimal risks, there is no guarantee that the final product will continue to be safe. Since manufacturers operate at or beyond the fringes of the law, their production process is unlikely to be highly regulated or intensely supervised. Inconsistencies in the process may lead to different final products or variable potencies.

Emerging drug manufacturers appear to be in a perpetual battle with policymakers and law enforcement. The reaction to each other's efforts appears to have created a complex "cat and mouse" dynamic. The pattern involves the shadow industry marketing a legal or quasi-legal product, policymakers expressly banning it, the shadow industry then switching to a new product that skirts the ban, and subsequent cycles of bans and replacement products. We refer to this continuous progression within the emerging drug industry as the "regulate and reformulate game." Perhaps no better example of the "regulate and reformulate game" exists than the recent history of synthetic cannabinoids in the USA. The manufacturers of synthetic marijuana products appear to be continually tweaking their products and manipulating psychoactive compounds to stay a step ahead of the law.

Early products marketed as synthetic marijuana under trade names such as Spice and K2 included benign plant material that had been combined with a psychoactive compound such as JWH-018 (Vardakou et al. 2010). The USA quickly took action and banned JWH-018 along with four other psychoactive products identified in the products marketed as legal marijuana alternatives (JWH-073, JWH-200, CP-47 497, and CP-47 497 C8 homologue) in March 2011. Unfortunately, this legislation failed to include some psychoactive compounds that had similar effects. Manufacturers could easily switch to compounds such as JWH-398, JWH-250, HU-210 (Vardakou et al. 2010), JWH-122, JWH-175, JWH-307, JWH-176, JWH-018-D$_3$, and cannabi-cyclohexanol (ACMD 2009) without having to alter their market strategy, packaging, or fear legal repercussions. A more comprehensive policy was enacted 16 months later in July 2012, but compounds such as CP-55,950, AM-694, and Win-48,098 might still be utilized by manufacturers. James Capra, DEA Chief of Operations, summarized the regulate and reformulate game in a recent press conference:

> "These are the types of individuals, criminals that we're dealing with: as soon as we schedule, as soon as we make these things illegal, criminal organizations will go back and they change one molecule. One! One molecule! And it changes the entire drug! It changes the whole structure of the drug so the drug becomes legal and we're at it again. And that's the dynamic of what we're facing." (Project Synergy Press Conference 2013)

The challenges that this progression presents for law enforcement are thoroughly presented in Chap. 5, but it may also substantially increase health risks. We expect that initial products are, at best, marginally assessed for their negative health repercussions (and are more likely underevaluated prior to marketing and distribution). It could be that underground chemists are evaluating their product on themselves and/or with their personal networks, likely in a nonscientific or systematic way. Furthermore, those middlemen handling the product from the producer until it reaches retail may modify the product before reaching the end user. The replacement compounds that are slight alterations in order to avoid the law are, likely, even more inadequately researched and tried on fewer human subjects prior to distribution. The changing of a single molecule may successfully skirt the law, but it also has the potential to massively increase the risks associated with use. There is potential for manufacturers, in haste to retain or quickly reclaim their market share after a ban, to take shortcuts that have lethal consequences.

3.1.2 Distribution and International Issues

One of the greatest challenges with regulating emerging drugs is that they may cross several borders before reaching the consumer. As a result, regulators in the countries in which they are sold have no opportunity, or more importantly no legal right, to inspect the manufacturing process or ensure that a consistent product is produced. Similarly, when a product is primarily shipped into a new country and distributed there, any legal change in the consumer country will only indirectly affect the manufacturer. Rather than the manufacturing process being shut-down and having to start from scratch, that company can redirect its products to a different consumer nation or continue to export the product with new labeling. Their risks are still manageable in that case. Since manufacturers typically operate in the Far East or in developing countries with weak regulatory schemes and limited resources to enforce drug laws (Griffiths et al. 2010), their operations and violations of international policy are not a high priority for their governments. Similarly, those countries are likely to be slow to collaborate with the consumer countries on which their citizenry is profiting. The worst likely scenario for overseas manufacturers is that their illicit product is intercepted and seized. Even in that event, their assets in the producing country remain safe and they continue to profit from those shipments that avoid interdiction. After a ban, they have the opportunity to continue their operation at low risk and then only have a limited interruption when switching to a slightly altered formulation of the product.

Interestingly, some manufacturers legally operate in countries in which the substances are banned so long as they only sell their products to retailers in another country. Griffiths et al. (2010, p. 952) note: "Internet retailers of 'Spice' based in the Netherlands, for example, can supply 'Spice' products to other EU countries but not their own." Thus, the emerging drug issue cannot be remedied by countries solely focusing on their own domestic policy. While regulation may place obstacles in the paths of manufacturers and alter the desirability of some chemicals, those entrenched within a drug using culture will likely continue to seek out and obtain novel psychoactive substances as long as they are available as a result of other countries' mass production. As such, it is imperative that developed and developing nations cooperate to equitably manage drug production and regulation.

3.2   The Sale and Marketing of Novel Drugs

Newer and emerging drugs may be obtained in a number of ways. Unlike traditional drugs, which almost exclusively reach the end users through a black market network, many of today's newer drugs can be obtained through the same channel as most consumer products. Whether they are psychoactive substances that skirt regulation by being slightly different from existing substances, include banned compounds but claim legality, or are just so new that they have not yet been regulated by local or federal government, they often appear in "head shops," other retail outlets, and online. Activists are often concerned that the availability of psychoactive products through "legitimate" providers may create a false sense of safety among potential users. The following sections detail the routes through which users may obtain emerging drug. Each of these appears to be the source for at least some of the drugs reaching consumers. However, since many users simply report obtaining novel drugs through friends (Khey et al. 2008) and do not know where their friends initially got them, it is challenging to estimate the proportion of novel drug users getting products sold through each channel.

3.2.1   Over the Counter Retail Sales

Many Americans that have chosen to experiment with psychoactive substances have found them readily available at local shops and stores. Typically, the products are sold at "head shops" or tobacco retail establishments that also sell paraphernalia designed to be used for smoking marijuana under the guise that it is being marketed to tobacco enthusiasts. In addition, novel psychoactive substances have been (and are being) sold at tattoo parlors, independent gas stations, truck stops, stores selling sexual products, and other similar outlets. These locations would likely offer advice about how to use the product if it was still legal to use recreationally. This advice, of course, is potentially biased by the owners' and clerks' desire to sell products and those individuals' personal experiences. In situations where a product avoids legal bans when labeled as "not for human consumption," store employees may avoid offering insight and advice that would violate the law. These situations may be even more problematic in that consumers may not receive any information about the product prior to purchase. Some reports from law enforcement suggest that legal bans effectively remove the psychoactive substances from the store shelves (Stogner et al 2012), but others suggest that many retailers just move the product from above the counter to below it (NACS 2012).

3.2.2   Street Dealers and Black Market Distribution

It does not appear that many of the emerging drugs of today, including those that have recently been banned, reach consumers through an elaborate black market or street dealers, at least in the USA. This may simply be due to the novelty of the bans; a black market distribution system may take more time to develop than has passed since the more recent emerging drug restrictions (Stogner et al. 2012). It would, therefore, be inappropriate to claim that salvia, cannabinoids, and bath salts will remain excluded from street markets simply because they are not sold in that way immediately after their ban. Many of the emerging drugs of the past, such as MDMA or ecstasy, now reach consumers through a black market distribution system. For the most part though, it appears that emerging drug consumers obtain their desired product through a retail outlet, online source, or their peers as opposed to a street dealer.

However, this is not universal. In 2011, McElrath and O'Neill found that mephedrone users in Belfast reported greater reliance on street dealers after a ban was passed in the UK. Furthermore, these researchers found that the packaging of this emerging drug emulated street drugs after it fell into the hands of street dealers, perhaps calling into question the consistency of an already questionable product. Winstock et al. (2010) also reported that UK users now mainly buy the stimulant from street dealers. As such, they are paying approximately twice as much and have even fewer guarantees of safety, purity, or quality. It is unclear why differences exist in the ability for emerging drugs to penetrate the black market across nations and the timing of this shift. However, it may be due to the availability of other drugs like MDMA, of which mephedrone has been reported as an emerging drug substitute.

It seems, though, that only in rare cases or after a long period of time do street dealers and black market distributers handle the bulk of emerging drug sales. Those drugs that are highly reinforcing and lend themselves to psychological dependence are most likely to have a quickly developing black market. Of course, this would likely only occur if no suitable licit replacements existed, the drug was considered by users to be equal to or better than street drugs in the same pharmacological family (it was not initially only utilized because of its previous legality), and a requisite threshold of users existed.

As discussed previously, not all emerging drugs are removed from store shelves following a ban. Additionally, consumers may purchase new versions of the product, advertised to be legal, that actually still contain the same compound that was banned (Ayres and Bond 2012). Shadow industry corporations may be taking advantage of overburdened law enforcement agencies that cannot test every product being sold for each banned compound. Similarly, both retailers and consumers may be deceived by a product with banned compounds' claims of legality. Since the door remains somewhat open for more efficient and direct routes of obtaining emerging drugs following bans, street dealers may be deterred from handling a product for which most of the market is spoken for and which has lower profit margins compared to traditional street drugs (due to other sources being available).

3.2.3 Online Sales

Emerging drugs marketed as "legal highs" are clearly available for purchase on the Internet. What is less clear is how often the websites selling the drugs actually deliver them, whether their products contain what they advertise, and whether they are responsible for a sizable portion of the emerging drugs that reach users. Several studies have confirmed that psychoactive substances are at least sometimes delivered after online purchase (Davies et al. 2010; Nakajima et al. 2011; Uchiyama et al. 2009) and some users report getting them through online vendors. Thus, the Internet appears to be responsible for a portion of drug sales, but data collected from casual users both in the USA and abroad suggest that the majority did not obtain them in this way (Khey et al. 2008; Barratt et al. 2012).

As part of the more complete analysis of online emerging drug providers, Davies et al. (2010) ordered 26 products monthly for 6 months. They initially found them to be consistently shipped, but received fewer and fewer products as the experiment continued. This may indicate that companies migrate their active providers from website to website to avoid taxation or legal repercussions. Alternatively, it may simply mean that many start-up drug delivery operations close down without removing their webpage or ceasing to take payments. Upon chemical analysis, Davies et al. (2010) also noted that there was variability in the consistency of the products received. One-quarter of the products received more than once during the 6-month study had at least two different formulations. Thus, users could quite possibly have received a different drug even when ordering the same product from the same website just a short time later. Davies et al.'s (2010) analysis also failed to identify any psychoactive compound in some products (e.g., placebo) and only identified caffeine in others. It seems that individuals who order a product marketed as a "legal high" online may either not receive anything at all or receive something that is no stronger than a couple of cups of coffee. While psychoactive products are reaching users through online sources, it appears that ordering an emerging drug online, even prior to a ban, may not be a reliable or economically efficient way of obtaining the drug.

These findings seem to mirror recent studies focused on online purchases of abused pharmaceuticals that indicate the Internet is not as common a source of misused medications as initially feared (Inciardi et al. 2007; Cicero et al. 2008). Cicero et al. (2008) reported that it was extremely difficult to get strong opioids online even after they spent more than US$ 2,000 at a variety of sites. As is the case for emerging drugs and novel highs, adolescents are much more likely to get pharmaceuticals to abuse through friends and family members (Boyd et al 2006; McCabe and Boyd 2005). Inciardi et al. (2007) found in a survey of prescription drug abusers admitted for treatment, that less than 5 % obtained medications from online sites. The authors note, though, that this sample is limited to heavier users since they are those either seeking, or have been forced to seek, treatment. Thus, a wider margin of modest to moderate recreational drug users may have success obtaining the quantities, types, and potencies they desire online while these heavy users may find it challenging to get what they desire from a site. In addition, a larger portion of the medications that the participants in this survey used may have been from online source, but purchased by a distributer rather than the end users.

Though salvia (Dennehy et al. 2005), cathinones (Davies et al. 2010), cannabinoids (Nakajima et al. 2010; Uchiyama et al. 2009), and piperazines (Davies et al. 2010) appear to have been readily available before bans and have remained available afterwards, these emerging substances should not be labeled "Internet drugs" any more than opioids and other pharmaceuticals. They may be purchased online, but they are not defined by their online status. Once again, research suggests that online providers are not the leading source of emerging drugs that reach users (Stogner et al. 2012; Khey et al. 2008).

In some instances, websites have specifically advertised that their formulation remained legal after a ban and others promoted new formulations. Despite these advertisements, they may not have actually altered their formula or effectively skirted legal restrictions. Ayres and Bond's (2012) analysis of psychoactive compounds marketed as "legal highs" indicated that newer products and products with new packaging often contain the same substances that were in previous generations and widely banned. It appears that the same compounds are often simply put into new packaging with new names to convince users, and perhaps even local law enforcement, that their purchase is legal. Given that online corporations often operate overseas, the consumer bears the legal risk from the seller's fraud.

Along with these traditional webspaces, there are a series of hidden web addresses that users with advanced knowledge can access to purchase novel drugs, illicit drugs more broadly, as well as other gray/black market products. These underground Internet addresses are collectively known as "the dark net." Very little is known about this underground marketplace and it is unclear the amount of emerging drugs that are bought and sold through this method.

3.3   The Role of the Internet in the Spread of Emerging Drugs

While the apparent availability of emerging drugs for purchase online has caused significant concern, many groups seem to be more worried about the potential negative influence of drug-promoting websites and social media postings. Although the Internet has proven to be a useful tool in education, the central fear seems to be that it may be teaching adolescents incorrect information about drugs and promoting what is typically considered deviant behavior. Numerous studies have described the plethora of information promoting drug abuse in general, detailing ways that substances can be abused, and discussing means of avoiding law enforcement (Boyer et al. 2005; Schifano et al. 2006). Many of these websites can be characterized as prodrug (e.g., Erowid.com) and are viewed by several million people each year. This, of course, does not guarantee that they are having an effect on attitudes and patterns of use—an important empirical question yet to be answered by extant research.

Mainstream researchers point out that many of these sites, like Erowid.com, include claims from pseudoscientists and enthusiasts that underestimate risks and give poor advice (Brush et al. 2004). This inaccurate information often appears factual, and many Internet users may not be able to distinguish those sites that are legitimate from those that are not (or even which portions of contributions on each site are legitimate as many of these sites' content is user-driven). One of the more popular features of many drug websites is their drug forum where users recount their experiences and opinions. As is the case with most online information, these postings are at best minimally vetted and should be viewed with heavy skepticism. As users and nonusers alike are prone to sensationalize and boast about exciting experiences to gain the attention of others, *all* forums are problematic if viewed without skepticism.

Prior studies have attempted to determine the proportion of information about drugs that is blatantly incorrect, but it is more relevant to determine how often and to what degree individuals believe incorrect information and lack the correct information. Several studies have explored how frequently information on the Internet is accepted as factual (Metzger et al. 2003; Flanagin and Metzger 2000; Johnson and Kaye 1998), however, most of those studies have focused on the perceived credibility of information about current events or political issues rather than substance abuse.

Case studies have identified users who claimed information on websites altered their use (Brush et al. 2004; Boyer et al. 2005). Other than these types of isolated reports, there is little evidence supporting the notion that viewing prodrug sites leads to altered views, initiation of use, or increases in use. Brewer (2003) attempted to fill this void by using an experimental design to determine to what degree Internet searching could affect attitudes toward using club drugs. In this study, 186 college students were assigned to spend 40 min searching for information on club drugs or were placed in a control group searching for information on an unrelated topic. Searching for information online increased knowledge about both ecstasy and speed in those who had not previously used drugs. Brewer (2003) also found that searching for this information led students to see greater benefits in using both of these club drugs, but this did not alter intention to use in the future.

To be certain, the information on the Internet has likely little effect on traditional street drug sales and use among those living in poverty since this segment of the population is unlikely to have sufficient access to technology (Cunningham et al. 2006). Thus, novel drugs seem to be a particular focus of this Internet-drug panic. Reports have implicated the Internet as the key provider of emerging drug information and facilitator of related curiosity (Hoover et al. 2008). However, we consider these concerns to be an overestimation given extant research, including our own efforts. The fear of emerging drug information on the Internet is based on what *could be* influencing behavior, but we suggest focusing our attention on what *is actually* influencing behavior. Very few users of emerging drugs cite the Internet as their main source of emerging drug information and few first learned of a drug online (Khey et al. 2008). Research suggests that friends and other contacts seem to be the primary providers of information and access to the substances. The Internet may be used to explore and gather information about emerging drugs after an individual hears of a new psychoactive substance, but it does not appear to typically be the original or primary source of information. They may use it as a tool to help locate a drug source, learn how to modify a pharmaceutical, or simply use a "pill lookup" to determine whether a pharmaceutical can be used to get high. Overall, it appears that while the public *perceives* that the Internet facilitated the spread of some emerging drugs, that information was *actually* conveyed through peers as is the case for more traditional drugs and that it *may assist* in behaviors chosen based on offline factors.

It is also pertinent to keep in mind that a communication tool should not be only viewed for its potential negative influences. Just as the social importance and impact of other information outlets such as television and newspapers is linked to content, the utility of the Internet as related to emerging drugs is tied to the quality of the available content. The Internet, particularly social media, has been successfully utilized in a variety of public health campaigns whose methodologies can be applied to emerging drug issues. However, we stress that communication efforts will be most successful when they are nonbiased and avoid over sensationalizing the issue. Just as rational readers reject blatantly biased prodrug information, they are likely to ignore unbelievable and excessively dramatic messages that promote abstinence. The US Navy's outlandish video related to bath salts (US Navy 2013) and Washington D.C.'s campaign that connects synthetic cannabinoid use to zombies (K2/Zombie DC 2013) may be two such examples.

3.4 Explaining Emerging Drug Use

Though it is clear that the Internet is not primarily responsible for the increasing numbers of novel drug users, the true culprit is not so easily identified. Emerging drug use may be linked to the same factors that influence more traditional drug use. If that is the case, then societal forces that effectively encourage (or curtail) traditional drug use should similarly affect emerging drug use. Thus, findings from previous generations of drug research should still be applicable to emerging drugs. As there is still substantial debate related to causes of individuals' drug use and the most effective interventions, this hypothesis remains challenging to assess and evaluate. Alternatively, many of the emerging drugs may not have their own distinct place in society. They may simply be substitutes for more desirable or more routinely used psychoactive substances chosen because of their availability or legal status. Finally, use of an emerging drug that is currently legal may be a developmental milestone in moderately deviant groups. That is, using the newest emerging drug may be somewhat of a rite of passage that adolescents feel pressure to complete in order to feel that they have completely fulfilled the expectations and matched the experiences of their peers. The following three sections address each of these alternatives presenting traditional theories of drug use as related to emerging drugs, novel drugs as replacements for banned substances, and emerging drugs as a social milestone.

3.4.1   Traditional Explanations of Drug Use

The differential use of drugs is typically attributed to one of three general sources: biological differences, psychological variation, or sociological forces (Goode 2008). The biological perspective typically attributes susceptibility to drug use to biological differences that cause some individuals to differentially respond to psychoactive substances. These differences yield higher levels of positive behavioral reinforcement and, thus, greater potential for dependencies after initiation use. This perspective may have greater utility for explaining why some individuals that are prescribed pharmaceuticals have a more difficult time ceasing use than others. But, it is at best marginally helpful in explaining novel drug use since habitual use is rare and it is unlikely that experimenters expect that the drugs will correct any preexisting metabolic imbalance. More recent work in this area has centered on determining whether genetic polymorphisms moderate reactions to stressful situations and traumatic life events (for an overview see Beaver 2009). However, there is no work of which we are aware that has explored gene-environment interactions as predictors of novel drug use.

Psychological theories of traditional drug use place more focus on the degree that substance-using behavior is reinforced either by the direct effect of the drug, the indirect repercussions of the use, or other factors (McAuliffe and Gordon 1975). Put most simply, this cluster of explanations considers the euphoria or high experience and the avoidance of withdrawal to be major motivating factors. Other psychological explanations suggest that drug use is linked to individuals supplementing "inadequate personality" types and still others explain drug use as the result of psychological traits that influence an array of poor decisions. Overall, it seems like the idea of reinforcement may assist in explaining the lack of habitual use of some novel substances more than it aids in explaining experimentation and initial use. Many of the emerging drugs, *Salvia divinorum* being an excellent example, have effects that the majority of users view as unpleasant (Stogner et al. 2012). This is likely the basis for most users failing to progress to habitual use. While it could be that initiation and experimentation with novel drugs are closely tied to expectations of positive reinforcement (i.e., how good the high will be), there is no evidence currently supporting that hypothesis. We expect that sociological explanations are more suited for this undertaking.

One of the most influential theories of behavior under the sociological perspective umbrella is Akers' social learning theory (Burgess and Akers 1966; Akers 2009). This theory has consistently and effectively been utilized to explain the initiation of drug use, habitual use, abuse, and cessation. Akers' social learning theory specifies four constructs linked substance use and other potentially negative behaviors. He (2009) argues that substance use is influenced by past rewards and punishments, expectations of future social and nonsocial rewards and punishment (differential reinforcement), perceptions of the appropriateness of substance use (definitions), exposure to substance users (differential association), and access to substance using models (imitation). Social learning's empirical support as related to drugs typically dwarfs that of competing theories (Akers 2009; Pratt et al. 2010; Warr 2002) and is useful whether the substance is legal (Krohn et al. 1985; Akers et al. 1989) or illegal (Akers and Cochran 1985; Akers et al. 1979). Social learning theory may have particular utility for novel drug use given that most are consumed in the presence of peers and peers seem to be the overwhelming source of novel drug information (Khey et al. 2008). At present only one study has explicitly utilized social learning theory constructs as predictors of emerging drug use, but that study (Miller et al. 2011) found strong support for the Akers' arguments.

A second leading criminological explanation of drug use is found within the work of Gottfredson and Hirschi (1990). They argue that all deviant and antisocial behavior, including drug use, can be linked to a single trait: low self-control. They suggest that self-control is not developed in the absence of appropriate parenting and that it influences most life decisions. Those without adequate self-control, according to Gottfredson and Hirschi (1990), are more likely to experiment with substances. Research does support the tenets of their theory and strongly connect low self-control or impulsivity to drug use more generally (Baron 2003; Connor et al. 2009; Smith and Crichlow 2012) and specifically emerging drug use (Miller et al. 2009), but in an emerging drug study that included both social learning and self-control variables, social learning variables were identified as being most closely connected to emerging drug use (Miller et al. 2011).

The majority of other leading individual-level sociological explanations of drug use and deviance appear to have less utility for novel and emerging drugs, particularly those that remain legal. While some drug use may be affected by the label applied to an individual by society (Becker 1953), stress (Agnew 1992), or weak connections to society (Hirschi 1969), no studies that gathered data from emerging drug users suggest that life stress, a deviant label, or weak bonds directly influenced the choice to initiate use. It does not appear that emerging drug use is a primary coping mechanism or a reaction to isolation (although it may be used as a substitute for a substance that is a primary coping mechanism).

In the last 20 years, there has been a renewed interest in criminological theory and research related to neighborhood structure and conditions. Large-scale studies with detailed measures of social and physical neighborhood conditions such as the Project on Human Development in Chicago Neighborhoods (PHDCN) have facilitated an outpouring of advances in macro-level theory. It seems to reason that neighborhood conditions may be closely related to the frequency of emerging drug use. Social and physical disorder as well as low collective efficacy likely increases the neighborhood level of general drug use (Sampson et al. 1997), but the relationship for emerging drugs may be more complex. A neighborhood that is extremely disorganized without any significant collective efficacy may tolerate heavy use of drugs and users may feel confident in their ability to avoid legal penalties. Since most users seem to prefer the traditional analogues of emerging drugs and because they are typically cheaper, this type of neighborhood may see heavy traditional drug use, but low emerging drug use. Emerging drug use may actually be more common in a moderate or moderately-low quality neighborhood in which potential users are concerned about residents intervening to stop traditional drug use, but are somewhat confident that their use of novel drugs, both legal and newly illegal, will not elicit a community response. Additionally, given that emerging drugs are often sold at "head shops," tattoo parlors, and independent gas stations while they are still legal (Fass et al. 2012), the use of emerging drugs is also likely linked to the number of these establishments in the community and their proximity to the neighborhood. We are unaware of any study that contrasts the relationships between neighborhood-level factors and traditional drug use to those for emerging drug use, but expect that this avenue of inquiry would be particularly rewarding and advance our understanding of emerging drug use.

3.4.2 Emerging Drugs as Replacements for Banned Substances

While a handful of drugs that at some point in the last 30 years could be labeled as novel or emerging are truly unique and cannot be easily likened to existing drugs of abuse (e.g., MDMA in the 1990s), the majority are viewed as replacements, alternatives, or substitutes for a more traditional drug. For example, users have referred to synthetic cathinones, which are marketed as bath salts, as "legal cocaine" and "legal methamphetamine" (Spiller et al. 2011), and synthetic cannabinoids are intended as a substitute for marijuana (Auwarter et al. 2009). Many have demonstrated that use of emerging drugs is most common among those that had previously used its more traditional analogue (Stogner and Miller 2013; Hu et al. 2011), but this does not necessarily implicate that emerging drugs are being used as alternatives in all cases. It may be that the overlap between a traditional drug and an emerging drug is simply due to the same factors influencing both. Several reports suggest that traditional marijuana remains more common and more highly desired than synthetic cannabinoids (Vandrey et al. 2012; Johnston et al. 2013; Stogner and Miller 2013) so it is doubtful that users perceive it to be a *superior* substitute. Thus, the role of an emerging drug as a substitute can be linked to a variety of factors.

Most likely when an individual chooses an emerging drug as a substitute for a drug they already desire, they are basing their decision on avoiding one of the potential negative repercussions of using the traditional analogue. They may choose a "legal high" to avoid the risk of identification and citation by law enforcement or regulators (e.g., Department of Transportation (DOT) drug screens for commercial drivers, train conductors, and pilots). The deterrence or rational choice perspective within the field of criminology suggests that decreased perceptions of legal risks would likely be linked to higher rates of use. Put more simply, potential users may sometimes choose the option that involves the least risk. The different risk potential in the late 2000s and early 2010s may have shifted some use from marijuana to synthetic cannabinoids, for example, but this shift was likely limited due to the differences in cost, loyalty to previously used strains, and perceptions that synthetic cannabinoids did not have as pleasurable an effect. Similarly, the relatively low risk of arrest for recreational marijuana users may have prevented many from feeling that they need to consider an alternative with reduced risk. Future research should evaluate whether fewer marijuana users experimented with synthetic cannabinoids in jurisdictions that have weak enforcement of marijuana laws.

Those under continuous surveillance for a subset of psychoactive drugs (e.g., community corrections, drug courts, and DOT drug testing regimens) may feel more pressure to choose emerging drugs as a substitute to get high without the fear of detection. In fact, even if a novel drug is already banned, users may still choose to use it as an alternative drug due to the expectation of a reduced likelihood of a positive drug screen (Vandrey et al. 2012). This line of thought may be one of the reasons that synthetic cannabinoid use is often connected to populations that undergo routine drug tests. Many anecdotal and academic reports suggest that use is higher in groups such as the military, probationers, and athletes that are tested for traditional drugs on a regular schedule or are selected for random screens. Additionally, some drug users may prefer to purchase products online or from a store as opposed to going through the hassle of locating a dealer even if the price of the emerging drug exceeds the analogue's street cost (see Gunderson et al. 2012; Hendricks and Dang 2012). While the replacement argument has merit and likely explains some use of novel drugs, it is incomplete. For example, if all (or most) of emerging drug use were related to replacement, use would drastically decrease after a ban and inclusion in drug screens. The USA's experience with synthetic cannabinoids demonstrates that a ban does not effectively curtail use. Further, a recent study suggests that mephedrone was added to the "drug repertoires" of European club patrons rather than replacing other psychoactive substances (Moore et al. 2013). Thus, while some emerging drug use may be the result of substituting one drug for another, these drugs become more than a fill-in for traditional drugs.

3.4.3 Emerging Drug Use as a Deviant Social Milestone

As an alternative to the previously mentioned explanations of drug use, we suggest that use of a legal psychoactive substance may have become a social and developmental milestone within some youth subcultures. Trying one of the emerging drugs with a relatively lower perceived likelihood of harm (such as salvia or a cannabinoid) may be a rite of passage or an informal initiation mechanism. It seems that many users have little desire to continue use even before their first experience and some may not desire the drug's effects at all. They use the drug just to try it, to see what the experience is like, and to simply have the experience. Their ability to honestly say that they have used the novel drug (or "a" drug) may be more important to them than the actual use of the drug. Their use may be influenced by the desire to have an experience that they perceive their peers have all had (Miller et al. 2013). To be clear, we do not hypothesize that experimentation is part of a formalized initiation process or driven by intense peer pressure. We suspect that it is more so motivated by individuals wanting to connect and share similarities with their peers. This may help to explain the use of those drugs that do not serve as true analogues of more traditional drugs or have strongly desired effects.

In many ways, the current generation of youth chooses to define itself through postings of videos, comments, and, more generally, by access to social media. They not only describe positive information and life successes online, but engage in proliferating and advertising as well as connecting with one another through what we can only label as the "spectacle of the stupid." Because humorous outcomes are more entertaining and adolescents often quantify the value of an experience in terms of "likes" and "hits" to that experience's videos or summary, we have seen a massive outpouring of videos depicting odd behavior. Videos abound of teens getting sick after eating a teaspoon of cinnamon, chugging a gallon of milk, or consuming some other odd product. Similarly, there is no shortage of clips that include pointless stunts or violent kicks to soft tissue areas. Even television shows exist that celebrate these clips and inspire and encourage new "spectacles of the stupid." These spectacles may be part of the coming of age process with novel drug experimentation just being one of the forms it takes. Use of *S. divinorum,* the subject of the first case study in the following chapter, may be best explained in this manner since it lacks a true analogue among traditional street drugs and is not strongly reinforcing. The typology of salvia users contained within that section argues that much salvia use can be attributed to these motives.

References

Advisory Council on the Misuse of Drugs. (2009). Consideration of the major cannabinoid agonists. Retrieved from https://www.gov.uk/government/publications/acmd-report-on-the-major-cannabinoid-agonists.

Agnew, R. (1992). Foundation for a general strain theory of crime and delinquency. *Criminology, 30*(1), 47–88.

Akers, R. L. (2009). *Social learning and social structure: A general theory of crime and deviance.* New Brunswick: Transaction Publishers.

Akers, R. L., & Cochran, J. K. (1985). Adolescent marijuana use: A test of three theories of deviant behavior. *Deviant Behavior, 6*(4), 323–346.

Akers, R. L., Krohn, M. D., Lanza-Kaduce, L., & Radosevich, M. (1979). Social learning and deviant behavior: A specific test of a general theory. *American Sociological Review, 44,* 636–655.

Akers, R. L., La Greca, A. J., Cochran, J., & Sellers, C. (1989). Social learning theory and alcohol behavior among the elderly. *The Sociological Quarterly, 30*(4), 625–638.

Auwärter, V., Dresen, S., Weinmann, W., Müller, M., Pütz, M., & Ferreirós, N. (2009). 'Spice' and other herbal blends: Harmless incense or cannabinoid designer drugs? *Journal of Mass Spectrometry, 44*(5), 832–837.

Ayres, T. C., & Bond, J. W. (2012). A chemical analysis examining the pharmacology of novel psychoactive substances freely available over the internet and their impact on public (ill) health. Legal highs or illegal highs? *BMJ Open, 2*(4).

Baron, S. W. (2003). Self-control, social consequences, and criminal behavior: Street youth and the general theory of crime. *Journal of Research in Crime and Delinquency, 40*(4), 403–425.

Barratt, M. J., Cakic, V., & Lenton, S. (2013). Patterns of synthetic cannabinoid use in Australia. *Drug and Alcohol Review, 32*(2), 141–146.

Beaver, K. M. (2009). *Biosocial criminology: A primer.* Dubuque: Kendall/Hun.

Becker, H. (1953). Becoming a marihuana user. *American Journal of Sociology, 59*(3), 235–242.

Boyd, C. J., Esteban McCabe, S., & Teter, C. J. (2006). Medical and nonmedical use of prescription pain medication by youth in a Detroit-area public school district. *Drug and alcohol dependence, 81*(1), 37–45.

Boyer, E. W., Shannon, M., & Hibberd, P. L. (2005). The Internet and psychoactive substance use among innovative drug users. *Pediatrics, 115*(2), 302–305.

Brewer, N. T. (2003). The relation of Internet searching to club drug knowledge and attitudes. *Psychology and Health, 18*(3), 387–401.

Brush, D. E., Bird, S. B., & Boyer, E. W. (2004). Monoamine oxidase inhibitor poisoning resulting from Internet misinformation on illicit substances. *Clinical Toxicology, 42*(2), 191–195.

Burgess, R. L., & Akers, R. L. (1966). A differential association-reinforcement theory of criminal behavior. *Social Problems, 14*(2), 128–147.

Cicero, T. J., Shores, C. N., Paradis, A. G., & Ellis, M. S. (2008). Source of drugs for prescription opioid analgesic abusers: A role for the Internet? *Pain Medicine, 9*(6), 718–723.

Cohen, P. A. (2012). Assessing supplement safety—the FDA's controversial proposal. *New England Journal of Medicine, 366*(5), 389–391.

Conner, B. T., Stein, J. A., Longshore, D., & Stacy, A. W. (1999). Associations between drug abuse treatment and cigarette use: Evidence of substance replacement. *Experimental and Clinical Psychopharmacology, 7*(1), 64–71.

Cunningham, J. A., Selby, P. L., Kypri, K., & Humphreys, K. N. (2006). Access to the Internet among drinkers, smokers and illicit drug users: Is it a barrier to the provision of interventions on the World Wide Web? *Informatics for Health and Social Care, 31*(1), 53–58.

Davies, S., Wood, D. M., Smith, G., Button, J., Ramsey, J., Archer, R., & Dargan, P. I. (2010). Purchasing 'legal highs' on the Internet—is there consistency in what you get? *QJM, 103*(7), 489–493.

Dennehy, C. E., Tsourounis, C., & Miller, A. E. (2005). Evaluation of herbal dietary supplements marketed on the internet for recreational use. *The Annals of Pharmacotherapy, 39*(10), 1634–1639.

Fass, J. A., Fass, A. D., & Garcia, A. S. (2012). Synthetic cathinones (bath salts): Legal status and patterns of abuse. *The Annals of Pharmacotherapy, 46*(3), 436–441.

Flanagin, A. J., & Metzger, M. J. (2000). Perceptions of Internet information credibility. *Journalism & Mass Communication Quarterly, 77*(3), 515–540.

Ginsburg, B. C., McMahon, L. R., Sanchez, J. J., & Javors, M. A. (2012). Purity of synthetic cannabinoids sold online for recreational use. *Journal of analytical toxicology, 36*(1), 66–68.

Goode, E. (1989). *Drugs in American society.* New York: Knopf.

Gottfredson, M. R., & Hirschi, T. (1990). *A General theory of crime.* Stanford: Stanford University Press.

Griffiths, P., Sedefov, R., Gallegos, A. N. A., & Lopez, D. (2010). How globalization and market innovation challenge how we think about and respond to drug use: 'Spice' a case study. *Addiction, 105*(6), 951–953.

Gunderson, E., Haughey, H., Ait-Daoud, N., Joshi, A., & Hart, C. (2012). Spice and K2 designer drugs: Synthetic cannabinoid consumption among marijuana and tobacco users. *Substance Abuse, 33*(2), 201–201.

Hendricks, L., & Dang, Q. (2012). K2: Synthetic marijuana-A NEW dangerous drug. *National Forum Journal of Counseling and Addiction, 1*(1), 1–7.

Hirschi, T. (1969). *Causes of Delinquency*. Berkeley: University of California Press.

Hoover, V., Marlowe, D. B., Patapis, N. S., Festinger, D. S., & Forman, R. F. (2008). Internet access to Salvia divinorum: Implications for policy, prevention, and treatment. *Journal of substance abuse treatment, 35*(1), 22–27.

Hu, X., Primack, B. A., Barnett, T. E., & Cook, R. L. (2011). College students and use of K2: An emerging drug of abuse in young persons. *Subsancet Abuse Treat Prevention Policy, 6*(1), 16.

Inciardi, J. A., Surratt, H. L., Kurtz, S. P., & Cicero, T. J. (2007). Mechanisms of prescription drug diversion among drug-involved club-and street-based populations. *Pain Medicine, 8*(2), 171–183.

Johnson, T. J., & Kaye, B. K. (1998). Cruising is believing? Comparing Internet and traditional sources on media credibility measures. *Journalism & Mass Communication Quarterly, 75*(2), 325–340.

Johnston, L. D., O'Malley, P. M., Bachman, J. G., & Schulenberg, J. E. (2013). *Monitoring the Future national survey results on drug use, 1975–2012. Secondary school students (Vol. 1, p. 604)*. Ann Arbor: Institute for Social Research, The University of Michigan.

K2/Zombie DC. (2013). *K2 + U = Zombie*. Retrieved from K2ZombieDC.com. Accessed 27 Nov 2013.

Khey, D. N., Miller, B. L., & Griffin, O. H. (2008). Salvia divinorum use among a college student sample. *Journal of Drug Education, 38*(3), 297–306.

Krohn, M. D., Skinner, W. F., Massey, J. L., & Akers, R. L. (1985). Social learning theory and adolescent cigarette smoking: A longitudinal study. *Social Problems, 32*, 455–473.

McAulifre, W. E., & Gordon, R. A. (1975). Issues in testing Lindesmith's theory. *American Journal of Sociology, 81*(1), 154–163.

McCabe, S. E., & Boyd, C. J. (2005). Sources of prescription drugs for illicit use. *Addictive behaviors, 30*(7), 1342–1350.

McElrath, K., & O'Neill, C. (2011). Experiences with mephedrone pre-and post-legislative controls: Perceptions of safety and sources of supply. *International Journal of Drug Policy, 22*(2), 120–127.

Metzger, M. J., Flanagin, A. J., & Zwarun, L. (2003). College student Web use, perceptions of information credibility, and verification behavior. *Computers & Education, 41*(3), 271–290.

Miller, B. L., Griffin III, O., H., Gibson, C. L., & Khey, D. N. (2009). Trippin' on Sally D: Exploring predictors of Salvia divinorum experimentation. *Journal of Criminal Justice, 37*(4), 396–403.

Miller, B. L., Stogner, J., Khey, D. N., Akers, R. L., Boman, J., & Griffin III, & O., H. (2011). Magic mint, the internet, and peer associations: A test of social learning theory using patterns of Salvia divinorum use. *Journal of Drug Issues, 41*(3), 305.

Miller, B. L., Boman, J. H., & Stogner, J. (2013). Examining the measurement of novel drug perceptions: *Salvia divinorum*, Gender, and Peer Substance Use. *Substance Use & Misuse, 48*(1–2), 65–72.

Moore, K., Dargan, P. I., Wood, D. M., & Measham, F. (2013). Do novel psychoactive substances displace established club drugs, supplement them or act as drugs of initiation the relationship between mephedrone, ecstasy and cocaine. *European addiction research, 19*(5), 276–282.

Nakajima, J. I., Takahashi, M., Seto, T., & Suzuki, J. (2011). Identification and quantitation of cannabimimetic compound JWH-250 as an adulterant in products obtained via the Internet. *Forensic Toxicology, 29*(1), 51–55.

North American Herbal Incense Trade Association. (2013). Why are herbal incense products labled (sic) "Not for human consumption." http://keepitlegal.org/content/why-are-herbal-incense-products-labled-not-human-consumption.

Parker, M. A., Marona-Lewicka, D., Lucaites, V. L., Nelson, D. L., & Nichol, D. E. (1998). A novel (benzodifuranyl) aminoalkane with extremely potent activity at the 5-HT2A receptor. *Journal of Medicinal Chemistry, 41,* 5148–5149.

Pratt, T. C., Cullen, F. T., Sellers, C. S., Thomas Winfree Jr, L., Madensen, T. D., Daigle, L. E., & Gau, J. M. (2010). The empirical status of social learning theory: A metaâĿanalysis. *Justice Quarterly, 27*(6), 765–802.

Project Synergy Press Conference. (2013). U.S. customs and border protection office of public [press release]. Affairs – Visual Communications Division. Retrieved from http://www.dvidshub.net/unit/USCBP#.UjC4SH-8BSo#ixzz2ebvWmohF.

Sampson, R. J., Raudenbush, S. W., Earls, F. (1997). Neighborhoods and violent crime: A multilevel study of collective efficacy. *Science, 227*(5328), 918–924.

Schifano, F., Deluca, P., Baldacchino, A., Peltoniemi, T., Scherbaum, N., Torrens, M., & Ghodse, A. H. (2006). Drugs on the web; the psychonaut 2002 EU project. *Progress in Neuro-Psychopharmacology and Biological Psychiatry, 30*(4), 640–646.

Smith, T. R., & Crichlow, V. J. (2012). A cross-cultural validation of self-control theory. *International Journal of Comparative and Applied Criminal Justice,* (ahead-of-print), 1–19

Spiller, H. A., Ryan, M. L., Weston, R. G., & Jansen, J. (2011). Clinical experience with and analytical confirmation of "bath salts" and "legal highs" (synthetic cathinones) in the United States. *Clinical Toxicology, 49*(6), 499–505.

Stiff Nights. (2013). Does stiff nights work? Retrieved from http://www.male-enhancement-review.org/stiff-nights/.

Stogner, J. M., & Miller, B. L. (2013). Investigating the 'bath salt' panic: The rarity of synthetic cathinone use among students in the United States. *Drug and alcohol review.*

Stogner, J., Khey, D. N., Griffin, O. H., Miller, B. L., & Boman, J. H. (2012). Regulating a novel drug: An evaluation of changes in use of Salvia divinorum in the first year of Florida's ban. *The International Journal on Drug Policy, 23*(6), 512–521.

The Association for Convenience and Fuel Retailing (NACS). (2013). The Association for convenience & fuel retailing. Retrieved from http://www.nacsonline.com/Pages/default.aspx

Uchiyama, N., Kikura-Hanajiri, R., Kawahara, N., & Goda, Y. (2009). Identification of a cannabimimetic indole as a designer drug in a herbal product. *Forensic Toxicology, 27*(2), 61–66.

United States Navy Medicine. (2013). Bath salts: It's not a fad . . . it's a nightmare. Retrieved from http://www.med.navy.mil/pages/spice.aspx.

U.S. Attorney's Office. (2013). Office of the United States Attorneys. Retrieved from http://www.justice.gov/usao/az/press_releases/2013/PR_07222013_Lane.html

U.S. Department of Justice (2011). Synthetic cathinones (bath salts): An emerging domestic threat. URL: http://www.justice.gov/archive/ndic/pubs44/44571/44571p.pdf. Accessed 27 Nov 2013.

Vandrey, R., Dunn, K. E., Fry, J. A., & Girling, E. R. (2012). A survey study to characterize use of spice products (synthetic cannabinoids). *Drug and alcohol dependence, 120*(1), 238–241.

Vardakou, I., Pistos, C., & Spiliopoulou, C. (2010). Spice drugs as a new trend: Mode of action, identification and legislation. *Toxicology letters, 197*(3), 157–162.

Warr, M. (2002). *Companions in crime: The social aspects of criminal conduct.* Cambridge: Cambridge UP.

Wiley, J. L., Marusich, J. A., Huffman, J. W., Balster, R. L., & Thomas, B. F. (2011). Hijacking of basic research: The case of synthetic cannabinoids. *Methods Report (RTI Press), 2011*

Winstock, A., Mitcheson, L., & Marsden, J. (2010). Mephedrone: Still available and twice the price. *The Lancet, 376*(9752), 1537.

Chapter 4
Case Studies of Emerging Drugs: Salvia, Bath Salts, and Bromo-DragonFly

In order to offer more insight into the novel and emerging drug phenomenon, a series of case studies are presented in the following pages that intricately explore the recreational use, media coverage, and regulation of three emerging psychoactive substances with diverse effects and unique histories. First, a short-acting dissociative plant in the mint family, *Salvia divinorum,* is described as an example of an extant drug that somewhat suddenly became linked to recreational use after the natural product was chemically enhanced, mass produced, and packaged for retail sale by a handful of organizations. This drug is also an excellent example of state-led drug regulation as opposed to federal oversight. Second, the chapter examines the appearance of psychoactive synthetic stimulants marketed as "bath salts." This category of substances received significant media attention and was quickly scheduled at the federal level in most countries. Finally, we present the recreational use of a recently synthesized research chemical that has yet to become a widespread drug of abuse. Bromo-DragonFly is a powerful and long-acting hallucinogen when taken recreationally.

4.1 Case Study 1: Salvia divinorum

Salvia divinorum, or commonly referred to by users and law enforcement by its genus name "salvia," has emerged as a new drug of concern in the last decade in the USA. Salvia has also been called the "diviner's sage," "magic mint," and "Sally D" and may be referred to by some as Purple Sticky, the name of a popular brand of fortified salvia product. Its use as a psychoactive drug, however, is far from a new phenomenon and likely preceded colonization of the Americas. Salvia is a naturally occurring plant in certain regions of Mexico, but it is considered an emerging drug since it is now being altered, marketed, transported, and administered in new ways and is reaching a larger base of potential recreational users.

D. N. Khey et al., *Emerging Trends in Drug Use and Distribution,*
SpringerBriefs in Criminology 12, DOI 10.1007/978-3-319-03575-8_4,
© Springer International Publishing Switzerland 2014

4.1.1   Historic Use of Salvia

Gordon Wasson authored one of the first academic references to salvia as a psychoactive drug in 1962. Wasson and colleagues had been annually exploring the Oaxaca region of Mexico throughout the previous decade to investigate the natives' use of psychoactive mushrooms in religious ceremonies. During their investigations, they learned of a plant occasionally used for its psychoactive properties when hallucinogenic mushrooms were unavailable. Wasson (1962, p. 77) reported that the Mazatec Indians considered salvia, referred to as *ska Pastora* in Mazatec culture, a "less desirable substitute" to mushrooms, but that they took some effort in cultivating the plant.

Within the Mazatec Indian culture, salvia was administered to the unhealthy by a *curandero* (a shaman or folk healer). In a way, salvia was a diagnostic tool that they believed could help determine the source of an illness. Wasson (1962) reported that the Mazatec Indians believed that an individual that drinks water containing the leaves would reveal the source of their malady during the ensuing semi-delirious state. As such, friends and family would observe the individual while they were under the influence and listen to their comments. Its use in this form led to salvia being referred to as the "diviner's sage."

4.1.2   Modern Salvia Use

The use of salvia did not appear to extend much beyond this form until the 1990s and then was only rarely consumed by recreational drug users (Appel and Kim-Appel 2007). Recreational users would choose to smoke dried leaves rather than drinking a water-based salvia mixture or holding leaves in one's cheek as was the custom in Mazatec religious and healing ceremonies. Additionally, recreational users often purchase modified salvia products in which the concentration of salvinorn A (the active ingredient) had been artificially increased through a modified growing process or the leaves being chemically impregnated with its own extract after being harvested.

When salvia is smoked using a tobacco or marijuana pipe, users experience a relatively short, but very potent high. The typical high from smoking lasts fewer than 30 min (Prisinzano 2005; González et al. 2006). Some recreational users choose to chew the leaves and experience a more "subtle" version of the plant's effects. When administered in this way, the salvia's effects, although weaker, can last an hour or more (Baggott et al. 2004). Salvia users most frequently report disorientation and an intense dissociative sensation that almost immediately follows the administration (Prisinzano 2005; González et al. 2006). Other reports seem to liken salvia's effects to those of LSD claiming mystical insights, psychedelic visual distortions, hallucinations, and mood alterations (Zawilska and Wojcieszak 2013), but these appear to be far rarer. Loss of consciousness and out-of-body experiences have also been associated with salvia use (González et al. 2006).

Initial reports in the USA suggested that salvia use was rare and sporadic, but did note that it might become a problematic drug in the future. In 2003, the Drug Enforcement Administration (DEA) did not have cause to believe that salvia was likely to become a club drug and decided to label it a "drug of concern" rather than scheduling it. At that time, they suggested that its use in the USA was and would continue to be limited to adolescents and young adults that regularly shop at "head shops." These outlets are likely a source of information for potential salvia users and later studies (i.e., Khey et al. 2008) would implicate them as a major source of recreational salvia. Internet searches for "legal high," "herbal high," or "safe legal high" would often return lists of websites selling salvia (Dennehy et al. 2005), and many offered different versions of their product with different concentrations of salvinorin A, the psychoactive compound responsible for the plant's effects. However, as previously mentioned, Internet purchasing does not appear to serve as a substantial source for users to acquire emerging drugs, including salvia (Khey et al. 2008).

4.1.3   Media Coverage and Regulation of Salvia

Much of the focus on salvia in the mid-2000s can be attributed to its label as a "legal high," arguably the first of its breed in the USA. The legal availability of salvia drew the interest of concerned groups while media outlets easily gathered the attention of the public by describing salvia as a scary new drug right at children's fingertips. In fact, initial media coverage may have actually spread curiosity about salvia among adolescents and young adults and facilitated increased experimentation during this time.

Salvia-focused media attention increased significantly when Delaware teen Brett Chidester committed suicide after having used the substance on January 23, 2006. Though his use of salvia may not have been the direct cause of his suicide, or even contributed to it, the media's portrayal of the event sparked a panic that led to some states banning salvia possession. The resulting Delaware legislation was even labeled "Brett's Law" (Griffin et al. 2008). Use of salvia, however, was not considered a cause of death in the Chidester case and was only retrospectively added after reports of previous salvia use were found in his personal journal (presumably due to political pressure). In the journal, Chidester described the drug as exposing him to new dimensions and feelings of emptiness. Chidester's autopsy did not find salvia in his system, but his family continues to attribute his death to salvia (Spring 2009). This may be an overwhelming oversimplification of complex behavior (Khey et al. 2008). In a situation like this where a young person dies at an early age, it may be easier to vilify a tangible product than unravel the full sequence of events that contributed to the saddening outcome. Being a relatively unknown and rare drug, salvia may have been ripe for vilification. Whereas the public would instantly deny that caffeine, tobacco, or marijuana was the leading cause of a suicide, they are unlikely to similarly question personal stories of a drug about which they know little. Where there are few users, high-profile cases may heavily influence public opinion. The family maintains a blog "Brett Chidester—Stolen Angel" to honor his memory and promote salvia regulation.

Prior to Chidester's death, Louisiana and Missouri were the only two states that had banned the use or possession of salvia. Whereas Louisiana enacted a specific law that prohibited growing, manufacturing, or distributing salvia in 2005, Missouri had simply added *S. divinorum* and salvinorin A to its list of controlled substances. A little over a month after Chidester's death, Delaware Senator Karen Peterson sponsored "Brett's Law" and the state classified salvia Schedule I just 14 weeks after the tragedy. By mid-2012, 27 states had scheduled salvia or passed a law that effectively banned possession while three others prevented its sale to minors (Stogner et al. 2012). Yet, salvia remains legal in most of the western and northeastern states. Thus, salvia regulation continues to be interesting in that the federal government has not acted and has completely left its legal status in the hands of state legislatures. This model is more consistent with drug regulation policies prior to the Second World War than the last several decades.

Years after the Chidester case, salvia once again received national attention when Jared Loughner opened fire with a semi-automatic handgun in Tucson, Arizona killing six people and injuring Congresswoman Gabrielle Giffords. Shortly after the horrific incident, the television news program Nightline reported on Loughner's recurrent use of salvia and introduced it as a possible cause of his delusions and concern with existential realities. Unlike Chidester's case, the Arizona shooting was not followed by a wave of states regulating salvia. Even Arizona refrained from modifying its policies. Though it may be simply the case of the states willing to regulate salvia, already having enacted legislation, it seems that the Loughner case was co-opted by those that favor gun control that quickly generated their own narrative to push the issues they believe in. In other words, for political gain (or other reasons), the Loughner shooting was tied to the issue of gun control. Therefore, access to the gun may have served the function of being the villain eliminating the need for salvia to serve that role. Salvia may have avoided further infamy since the tragic event had already been blamed on something. To be clear, it is likely that neither case was directly driven by salvia; the distinction is that the Chidester family and news outlets pushed the salvia connection more so than those covering the Arizona shooting. Regardless, each tragic event increased public awareness of salvia and depicted it in a negative light.

4.1.4 The Scope of Salvia Use

Initial reports of salvia use and its effects when smoked came from case studies or small samples of users (Bücheler et al. 2005; González et al. 2006). For example, González and his colleagues surveyed 32 admitted salvia users in Spain. Members of their sample were frequent users of other drugs, but fewer than half expected to use salvia regularly in the future. It appears that they viewed their experience as somewhat positive citing the euphoria and dissociation as pleasurable outcomes, but disliked the ensuing lack of control and unpleasant after-effects (González et al. 2006). While studies like this one and Baggott's web-based survey of users (Baggott et al. 2004) were helpful in understanding the perceptions of salvia, its effects, and its utility among those strongly involved with drug use in general, they could neither be used to estimate the prevalence or frequency of use in the population nor were they able to detail less frequent drug users' reaction to salvia. For these issues, randomized samples of the population (or select portions of it) are necessary.

Due to ease of access to subjects and the fact that drug use is common during the collegiate years, many early assessments of salvia use relied on samples of university students. James Lange and his colleagues were among the first to evaluate the prevalence of salvia use. They found that 4.4 % of students at a southern California university had used salvia and argued that males, whites, and individuals that use other drugs used salvia more often. Later, David Khey et al. (2008) found that only 22.6 % of University of Florida students had even heard of salvia, but that a third of these (6.7 % of the total sample) had used salvia in their lifetime. Their results further suggested that continued use of salvia was rare.

S. divinorum was added to the National Survey of Drug Use and Health (NS-DUH) in 2006. The NSDUH, sponsored by the Substance Abuse and Mental Health Services Administration (SAMHSA 2007), surveys 70,000 randomly selected individuals annually to provide national and state-level statistical information on drug use. According to the NSDUH in 2006, only 0.9 % of teens (12–17 years old) had ever used salvia and even fewer had used in the last month (0.1 %). These rates slowly grew over the next 4 years reaching 1.6 % in 2010. A larger portion of young adults (18–25 years old) reported use (3.6 % in 2006), but few older adults (26 and older) reported use (0.2 %). Adult salvia use also substantially increased between 2006 and 2010. In 2010, 8.8 % of young adults and 0.9 % of older adults reported ever using the substance. The past year and month rates suggest that the majority of those that have experimented with salvia do not continue to use over a long period of time. Recent findings from the NSDUH suggest that the prevalence of salvia use has been relatively stable since 2010 (SAMHSA 2012).

Salvia was not added to the USA's annual national study of high school students (Monitoring the Future [MTF]) until 2009, so the study has limited utility in tracking trends in use throughout the salvia's emergent period. It, however, will be helpful in tracking salvia trends once several years of data have been collected, and it also does help to clarify and confirm estimates from the NSDUH. Given that the average age of participants in its sample are older than that of NSDUH's youth subsample, it is not surprising that its estimates of salvia use are higher. The most recent MTF results noted that salvia use was reported by 1.4 % of 8th graders, 2.5 % of 10th graders, and 4.4 % of 12th graders. It also appears from the MTF data that fewer high school students view salvia as harmful as compared to normal drugs. This could be problematic and indicate that users overestimate the drug's safety. In MTF, data do suggest that use may be decreasing among youth. There was a statistically significant drop in reported salvia use between 2011 and 2012. Whereas approximately 3.6 % of students reported using in 2011, only 2.7 % reported the behavior in 2012. This decrease in use may be the product of increased legal controls or simply the substance falling out of favor.

While this text largely focuses on the USA, it should be noted that salvia has been used throughout the world and many countries encountered salvia use before the USA. For example, Spain (González et al. 2006), Italy (Pavarin 2006), and Switzerland (Giroud et al. 2000), all had issues with salvia before the first US state regulated the substance. Additionally, even though *S. divinorum* is native only to Mexico, it seems to be grown throughout the world. Most smoked salvia is adulterated or fortified in some way to increase its potency, but its base is still the organic plant. As early as the late 1990s, salvia was discovered in indoor marijuana-growing facilities in Switzerland (Giroud et al. 2000).

4.1.5   Salvia: An Internet Phenomenon?

Some early reports suggest that the spread of salvia use was largely facilitated by its prominence on the Internet (Hoover et al. 2008). A fear promoted by media outlets looking to capitalize on parents' and other concerned citizens' protective impulses was that children and teens would learn of salvia, discover its legality, purchase the drug, and learn how to use it from online webpages established to promote salvia use. There is no question that salvia was readily available online and that several websites were established promoting its use (Dennehy et al. 2005). Additionally, heavily trafficked drug user forums such as Erowid.org and Lycæum.org often offered positive reviews of the substance.

Valerie Hoover et al. (2008) completed a complex review of salvia's web presence over a 2-year period. They suggested that salvia was an ideal Internet drug because of its legality in some states, the public's limited awareness of its effects and dangers, its potency, and the ease of cultivation/manufacturing and, therefore, assessed salvia-related web content. Their research found that approximately 60 % of sites returned on Google and Yahoo! using the search term "*Salvia divinorum*" either offered to sell the substance or linked directly to a website that did. Over three-quarters promoted salvia use in some way and only 2 % classified it as a treatment or anti-drug. Further, this study indicated that many sites misinterpreted scientific evidence or interpreted the lack of scientific evidence on toxicity, health impairments, addictive potential, or other consequences as positive evidence of its safety. This implies that potential users, likely teens and young adults, may not appropriately question the pro-salvia arguments or realize that the limited evidence of toxicity does not equate to a confirmation of safety. Further, these researchers found that salvia-promoting sites are inconsistent in their analogies: Many likened it to a legal substitute to cannabis, others to hallucinogens, and still others (very inaccurately) to opioid analgesics.

Research on young adult populations suggests that friends played a much greater role in transferring information about salvia prior to scheduling than did the Internet. Very few respondents from general surveys reported learning of the drug online and less than 10 % reported ever purchasing it online (Khey et al. 2008). Friends were much more often the key source of information, and "head shops" were the overwhelmingly most common mode of acquisition. Additional evaluations of young adult populations suggest that friends continue to be the most common information source, and salvia was rarely purchased online (Stogner et al. 2012). It appears that while pro-salvia information is readily available on the Internet, it actually is used infrequently, viewed skeptically, or only used by young adults to supplement the information passed along by their friends.

Salvia's favorable reviews and availability on the Internet likely had little to do with its legality. While some users may have been motivated to post messages and create websites in order to assist with the continued legality of salvia, the most common motivations are likely profit. As most sites offered to sell salvia or were associated with a site that did, they profited from giving positive reviews of the product. The promotion of a psychoactive substance for sale online is certainly not linked to the legality of the drug. Numerous rogue pharmacies claiming to sell prescription opioids and other scheduled pharmaceuticals exist online. Similarly, sites claiming to legitimately sell pharmaceuticals but failing to require adequate prescriptions or meet pharmaceutical standards are common on the Internet. Thus, the issue of Internet drug promotion or sales is not linked to a drug's legal status or unique to salvia, but is a larger issue shared by many drugs. We must also consider that simply because a substance is being advertised and is available for purchase online does not mean that it will reach the consumer. These websites may be utilized only sparingly or rarely deliver the product after purchase. Investigations into illicit pharmacies have suggested that those sites frequently charge potential consumers for drugs that they never ship or deliver (Chandra and Cupps 2002). As these victims are violating the law, they are unlikely to report not receiving their expected shipments. In this case, sales of salvia to states in which it is banned may be more an issue of fraud than substance use.

The Internet has aided our understanding of salvia use in several ways as well. In addition to web-based surveys, academics have gathered a great deal of information online via YouTube. Many groups have recorded and posted videos of individuals using salvia. Lange and others completed a detailed systematic observation of these posted videos and significantly improved our understanding of the effects that the drug has on individuals in a nonclinical setting (Lange et al. 2010). Their assessment helped clarify the delay of symptom onset and duration of effects in a typical drug-use setting. They noted the frequency of symptoms such as hypo- and hyper-movement, speech impairment, excitation, fear, and overheating which suggests that clinical effects may be subtler than effects observed outside a laboratory.

4.1.6   Typology of Salvia Users

Academic and anecdotal evidence would suggest that salvia is used in different ways and in different contexts. It appears that most use, and most users, could be classified as one of three types. First, there are "experimental users." These individuals use once or twice when in the company of friends and do not progress to habitual use. The use of these individuals may have been facilitated by salvia's legal status (and continue to be facilitated in those states where it's legal), but use may have occurred regardless. Use of salvia may be a rite of passage in certain groups or be an informal type of hazing. Members of the group may persuade new members to use so that they can witness and laugh at their high. Additionally, it appears that some individuals enjoy having the experience of using salvia, but show little interest in using again. Thus, in a way it may be perceived as part of a checklist of risky behaviors to be completed as a young adult. These individuals likely view themselves as someone who has used salvia rather than a salvia user.

Another type of salvia use is connected to those more involved in drug use and the drug using culture. Those that consider marijuana or psychedelics as their primary drug(s) of choice are particularly likely to experiment with salvia. Salvia itself appears to be used not as a drug of choice, but as one drug among many that the individual uses. It is unlikely that salvia acts as any type of a gateway agent for these users. Their drug use is likely diverse and frequent, and they may even pride themselves in the number of drugs they have tried or their knowledge about drug use. Their use may have originated with seeing a new product in a "head shop" they frequented and the desire to remain current with "advances" in drug use. For them, salvia is just another piece of the drug puzzle. Much like the experimental salvia users, the "avid drug users" appear unlikely to advance to habitual or regular use although they may occasionally or intermittently use. Given that they are more likely to be identified as drug/salvia users and they frequent locations and websites associated with drug use, these users are likely overrepresented in focused samples (i.e., González et al. 2006; Baggott et al. 2004).

A very small subset of salvia users may progress to become "ritualistic users." Although this appears to be very rare, there are individuals who may select salvia as their drug of choice and define the dissociative experience produced by the substance as pleasurable. This group is likely to tie salvia use to its origins in mystic religions and use the substance (and other psychoactive drugs) as a form of meditation or self-exploration. The ritualistic user would be very knowledgeable about the effects of the drug and be most likely to use it in its traditional forms (chewed as a leaf or mixed into a drink). This group would likely not be deterred by the illicit status of salvia, but unlike avid drug users they are less likely to have drug-related problems given their more structured use.

If this typology accurately represents salvia users, the scheduling of salvia may have very limited utility. The avid drug users are likely to continue to desire and use salvia regardless of its legality just as they use other illicit drugs. The scheduling may make salvia more challenging to obtain, but these individuals would likely be motivated enough to expand their drug experiences that they would be willing to violate the law and navigate obstacles. Ritualistic use of salvia would likely be similarly unaltered. Since experimental users are likely to only use a limited number of times, scheduling salvia would have little effect on drug-related harms experienced by this group. Once the substance is scheduled, this type of individual may not ever use salvia. Members of this group may not be willing to go through the hassle of obtaining salvia given that more pleasurable drugs may be more easily obtained. However, given that salvia has not been directly linked to automobile accidents or short-term negative health outcomes, a small reduction in use likely has negligible benefits at best. However, if salvia is truly acting as a rite of passage or risky behavior for the sake of experience in young adult peer groups, it is possible that another more dangerous substance or behavior will fill this void. As noted by Stogner et al. (2012), due to it being minimally reinforcing, salvia's role may have simply run its course with individuals becoming less interested after its novelty wore off and newer drugs became available.

4.1.7 Lessons from Salvia Use in the USA

S. divinorum, as an emerging drug, is an interesting case. As it is typically viewed as less reinforcing and less pleasurable than other psychoactive drugs, it may never have become even remotely popular if "head shops" were not able to legally sell it and if media did not sensationalize it as a "legal high." However, as noted previously, salvia regulation may not be as useful as one would suspect. Additionally, salvia is an excellent example of how a long-existing substance can spark an emerging drug threat following enhanced manufacturing, marketing, and distribution. The case of salvia also provides evidence of how a single event, perhaps even only tangentially related to the drug, can significantly affect willingness to regulate and possibly more importantly, public perception. This model mirrors events that have heavily influenced perceptions of other drugs such as the act of attempted cannibalism that was (inaccurately) linked to "bath salts" in Florida in 2012. Finally, salvia's Internet presence may have been erroneously blamed for its spread in the mid-2000s. This case suggests that the presence of pro-drug websites may only be marginally important in comparison to peers.

4.2 Case Study 2: Synthetic Stimulants Called "Bath Salts"

The term "bath salts" has been used to refer to a diverse group of commercially produced synthetic stimulants that reached drug-using populations in the last decade. These stimulants were produced as drugs for the purpose of euphoria and increased energy. As previously mentioned and contrary to their tacit claims, these products were never intended as a bathing aid or even sold in stores specializing in bath products. Some forms were instead labeled as "stain removers," "insect repellent," "plant food," or even "ladybug attractant" to similarly bypass regulations, but the name bath salts is typically used by the law enforcement, the media, and users to collectively refer to synthetic stimulants marketed in this way.

Though some legitimate consumers of bathing aids may have been concerned after initial reports of bath salts as a psychoactive substance prior to bans, there was little chance of accidental purchase of psychoactive bath salts. Rather than being sold in major retail outlets and stores specializing in spa and bath aids, these synthetic stimulants were most commonly sold over the Internet and in "head shops," tattoo parlors, pawnshops, discount tobacco outlets, truck stops, and some independent gas stations (Fass et al. 2012; Spiller et al. 2011). Additionally, rather than having a soothing title as one would expect for a bath product, psychoactive bath salts were often labeled in a way that reflected their intense and stimulating effects: "Blitz," "Zoom," "Atomic," "Hurricane Charlie," "White Lightning," "Spark," "Charge+," "White Rush," and "Scarface." Though the fear that a person may accidentally purchase psychoactive bath salts may have contributed to public outrage at their initial legal status, it was unrealistic.

Substances falling into the category of bath salts likely contain one or more compounds that mimic the effect of cathinone, an amphetamine-like alkaloid found in leaves of the *Catha edulis* (khat) that naturally grows near the Red and Arabian Seas (Prosser and Nelson 2012). The compounds most commonly labeled as bath salts are Methylenedioxypyrovalerone (MDPV), mephedrone, methylone, 4-Methoxymethcathinone, and 4-Fluoromethcathinone, but products may also contain butylone, dimethylcathinone, ethcathinone, ethylone, or 3-fluoromethcathinone. These chemicals act as powerful central nervous system stimulants by inhibiting the reuptake of monoamine neurotransmitters. For example, MDPV primarily inhibits norepinephrine–dopamine reuptake (Westphal et al. 2009; Baumann et al. 2012; Lehner and Baumann 2013) while mephedrone mostly inhibits serotonin reuptake (Dybdal-Hargreaves et al. 2013).

4.2.1   *Bath Salts and the Body*

The typical use of bath salts occurs after the purchase of a packet of 50 mg or more of a white (sometimes tan or brown) powder that costs between US$ 25 and 50 (Fass et al. 2012). Most reports suggest that the most common route of administration is nasal insufflation (inhalation through the nose), but intravenous injection (likely after dissolving the powder in water) and ingestion also appear to be common (Murray et al. 2012). Additionally, there have been reports of bath salts being smoked (Wright et al. 2012), administered rectally (Khan et al. 2013), and taken sublingually (Coppola and Mondola 2011) but it is unknown how frequently, or even if, bath salts are utilized in each of these ways. The case reports offered by Winder et al. (2013) suggest that some brands can be smoked, but most melt or burn when heat is applied. The speed at which intoxication appears is, of course, linked to the form of administration, but even with ingestion, the effects peak in less than 2 h (Ross et al. 2011). Symptom onset is more rapid with other common forms of administration and the most notable effects last approximately 3–4 h (Fass et al. 2012).

As previously mentioned, bath salts' effects are more similar to cocaine, amphetamines, and methamphetamines than other drugs. Most users experience increased energy, heightened alertness, increased libido, and euphoria. Bath salts also increase blood pressure and heart rate, decrease appetite, and prevent sleep. Users may become agitated and anxious or develop muscle spasms and nosebleeds. Some experience untoward symptoms such as severe paranoia, panic attacks, delusions, and extreme hallucinations that have been linked to hazardous and unpredictable behavior. Further, while under the influence of bath salts, many individuals become aggressive, violent, and combative. As such, bath salt use presents a significant danger to both users and the general public. Hyperthermia is also common which may explain why some users remove their clothing after taking bath salts. In the most problematic instances, bath salts have driven liver failure, kidney failure, seizures, and death (Meyer et al. 2010; Schifano et al. 2011; Murray et al. 2012; Fass et al. 2012; Adebamiro and Perazella 2012).

Many users of bath salts re-dose during a single drug episode. That is, they administer more of the drug to intensify or extend the high (Coppola and Mondola 2011; Streur et al. 2011; Schifano et al. 2011). This is not unlike how users go on a "binge" or "run" with more common stimulants. Heavy users also may develop a tolerance to bath salts (Freeman et al. 2012). As with other stimulants, bath salt users also report symptoms associated with psychological dependence after ceasing long-term use. Those quitting use report fatigue, reduced energy, depression, anhedonia, anxiety, craving, and insomnia that continue for a long period of time after the last use (Winstock et al. 2011; Winder et al. 2013). However, as is the case with most drugs that are only used by a small portion of the population, most of the knowledge of bath salts' effects and potential for dependence is reliant on case studies and reports consisting of few users (Antonowicz et al. 2011; Penders and Gestring 2011). Additionally, the reported number of deaths may be an overestimate of deaths actually caused by bath salts since many involved multiple drugs (Prosser and Nelson 2012). However, a preponderance of reports link bath salts to problematic outcomes and suggest that it should receive greater attention than most other emerging drugs.

4.2.2   The Emergence of Bath Salt Use

In terms of bath salt use, the USA lagged behind Europe, Australia, and other parts of the world. Mephedrone, marketed as a bath salt, became increasingly popular in the UK during 2008–2009. Winstock et al. (2010) found that over 40 % of 2,295 visitors to a popular UK dance music website had used mephedrone. An overwhelming majority of these users had used it in the last month. This study also assessed MDPV use, but found it to be much rarer (1.9 %) in the sample. Dargan et al. (2010) explored use in a more representative sample of young adults (one thousand Scottish students) noting that 20.3 % had used at least once and 4.4 % used mephedrone on a daily basis. Additionally, a number of bath salt-related Swedish deaths were identified as early as 2009 (Gustavsson and Escher 2009). Further, over 14 % of urine samples from an Irish heroin treatment clinic were found to contain evidence of mephedrone (McNamara et al. 2010), and a Finnish study identified MDPV in 8.6 % of samples taken from individuals suspected of intoxicated driving (Kriikku et al. 2011). Several other studies also suggested that bath salts were being increasingly used in Europe (Brandt et al. 2011; McElrath and O'Neill 2011; Prosser and Nelson 2012).

Though the UK and many nearby countries regulated mephedrone in 2010, its use continued. Winstock et al. (2010) reported that 63 % of their UK sample of mephedrone users continued to use, but complained that the price had more than doubled as a result of the ban. Alternatively, Carhart-Harris et al.'s (2011) research suggests that the majority of these users at least reduced their use as a result of the ban. Several bath salt-related deaths were also reported in the UK, which confirmed its presence in the region (Fass et al. 2012).

Around the time the UK banned bath salts in 2010, use reached the USA (Spiller et al. 2011). Initially, the only clear evidence that bath salt use was becoming more frequent was an increasing number of calls to poison control centers focused on managing the effects of bath salts (Johnston et al. 2013) and it being identified in a handful of laboratories (DEA 2013). Several deaths had been attributed to the drug (Johnson 2011; Murray et al. 2012; Wright et al. 2012), and the media had announced several cases of suspected bath salt use, but Spiller and colleagues provided the first truly insightful look into US bath salt in 2011. They retrospectively reviewed 236 cases of bath salt intoxication reported to poison centers and identified common symptoms, results, and laboratory findings (Spiller et al. 2011). Though bath salts were first federally restricted in 2011, very little additional information is known about the extent of bath salt use in the USA. Questions about bath salts were added to the national Monitoring the Future study in 2012, and it was found that 0.8, 0.6, and 1.3 % of 8th, 10th, and 12th graders, respectively, had used bath salts at least once (Johnston et al. 2013). Stogner and Miller's (2013) later research noted that 1.1 % of a large collegiate sample had used bath salts in their lifetime.

One thing that does appear clear is that the main psychoactive compound in products marketed as bath salts in the USA is MDPV (Spiller et al. 2011). This is in contrast to European bath salts, which were primarily mephedrone or, less commonly, methylone. It is not clear whether this distinction was driven by convenience, avoidance of regulation, market forces, consumer preferences, or producers moving on from a product that had already been stigmatized in another country. That being said, the composition of bath salt products in a given country is likely to vary, as is their potency. As such, users cannot be confident that they are taking the same substance that they took in the past or had seen others take.

It appears that bath salt users are more entrenched in the drug using culture than those that experiment with previously mentioned novel drugs like salvia or synthetic cannabinoids. Most are males and have an extensive history of drug use or at the very least use other substances (Fass et al. 2012; Stogner and Miller 2013; Porrovecchio 2011). Many apparently experimented with bath salts as a replacement for cocaine or another stimulant due to supplies of the previously used drug becoming limited, to avoid legal repercussions, or to avoid a positive drug test (Karila and Reynaud 2011). It seems that bath salts are more of an alternate or replacement stimulant as opposed to the so-called gateway drug.

4.2.3 US Media and Cultural Panics Linked to Bath Salt Use

Beginning in 2011, several prominent reports of aggressive and bizarre behavior attributed to bath salt use initiated what might be labeled a minor modern drug panic. Many of the stories that reached the national stage may have been sensationalized, and each vilified bath salt use. Two major stories aired in April 2011. ABC News covered the overdose and death of a Florida bath salt user, and a military officer was involved in a murder-suicide. Sergeant David Stewart allegedly suffocated his 5-year-old son, led law enforcement on a high-speed chase, shot his wife, and took his own life under the influence of "bath salts" (ABC News 2011; ABC24 2011; Johnson 2011). This horrific act led many members of the public to fear not only the direct effects of bath salts but also being violently victimized by a bath salt user. A month later, a West Virginia man was arrested after he was found wearing women's lingerie in his bedroom with a goat that he had allegedly raped and killed (Sheridan 2011), and a man in Tennessee reportedly attempted to perform surgery on himself under the influence of "bath salts" (ABC24 2011). However, as *The Economist* (2012) noted, "few things command attention like a random act of cannibalism."

The panic reached a precipice in May 2012 when a naked Rudy Eugene cannibalistically attacked Ronald Poppo in Miami. Eugene, who removed both of Poppo's eyes and most of his nose during the attack, was shot and killed by police responding to the incident. His behavior was attributed to "bath salts" (Dahl 2012) despite later reports that indicated that Eugene did not have MDPV or synthetic cathinones in his system (Hiaasesn and Green 2012). Media outlets dubbed him the "Causeway Cannibal" and bath salts the "zombie drug." Even a year after the incident and after reports that Eugene had only used marijuana, the majority of the populace primarily associates bath salts with cannibalism. We interviewed numerous law enforcement officers, educators, and military personnel about their knowledge and opinions related to emerging drugs (not yet published). The overwhelming majority of those that had heard of bath salts linked it to the cannibalistic Miami attack when asked what they knew about the drug.

Bath salts continue to be linked to bizarre behavior. A month after the Miami incident, a naked Pamela McCarthy choked her 3-year-old before running into the streets of Munnsville, New York and attempting to strangle her dog. She died of cardiac arrest after a conflict with police that led to her being tasered (Nelson 2012). While McCarthy had a history of bath salt use and was likely under the drug's influence, there has been no indication of bath salt use by Jett McBride, the Tacoma man who while claiming to be Jesus drove his car into pedestrians and began assaulting them until stopped by Caleb "Kai the hitchhiker" McGillivary. The lack of confirmation that McBride was a bath salt user, however, did not keep the members of the media (such as former ESPN host Jim Rome) from making assumptions about McBride's substance use that may have further exacerbated concern over bath salts (Rome 2013).

Each of these incidents, and even more so, the group as a collective, fanned the flame of public outrage. Bath salts appeared to be a growing menace moving in terms of public awareness from unheard of to repeatedly causing unexpected and violent behaviors in less than 2 years. Even though their use is still somewhat rare, the media implied bath salt use had "exploded" (Roff 2012), "runs rampant" (Cross 2012), and even had hit "epidemic proportions" (Erickson 2011). This may have initiated or exacerbated the concern of the public that they were just starting to sense the initial effects of a bath salt outbreak. The forms of bizarre behavior reported may also have furthered public panic in that many people fear the unpredictable. While other psychoactive drugs cause them concern, they may take some comfort in knowing what happens after someone uses marijuana, LSD, or heroin. The nondrug using population is likely to know very little about an emerging substance like bath salts and fear the unknown. Similarly, in the absence of other information, they are likely to believe media reports that only focus on the most sensationalistic cases of bath salt use (or even sensational events that do not involve bath salts).

While the previous paragraphs should clearly present the opinion that bath salt coverage was inaccurate, sensationalized, and led to a misinformed population, readers should not infer that the reports and public concern failed to yield positive effects. As described in previous sections, MDPV, mephedrone, and other compounds labeled as bath salts are quite dangerous. Whether the public supported regulation because they inaccurately believed bath salts drove cannibalism or because they were well informed about its toxicity, link to violence, and potential for psychological dependence may be somewhat politically unimportant. In both circumstances, they support regulation and removal from store shelves. Ideally, voters and politicians should make the "right" decision for the "right" reasons, but implementing the "right" policy for the "wrong" reason is likely far better than taking no action at all or enacting problematic legislation. While regulation may not eliminate use, it would likely cause an increase in price (Winstock et al. 2010) and decrease in frequency of use (Carhart-Harris et al. 2011) as was reported in the UK.

4.2.4   Regulation of Bath Salts and Results

As use of bath salts in the UK preceded their use in the USA, it would be expected that the UK would ban mephedrone and other cathinone derivatives prior to the USA. They regulated them on April 16, 2010 under the 1971 Misuse of Drugs Act and the Republic of Ireland soon followed suit. Other European countries followed as did more than half of the US states. The US Federal Government placed a 1-year ban on MDPV, mephedrone, and methylone in the fall of 2011. This temporary emergency scheduling was chosen to allow the DEA time to collect data and evaluate the substances before placing them in a schedule, which may limit scientific research or interfere with individual liberties. In July of 2012, President Obama signed the Synthetic Drug Abuse Prevention Act of 2012 and the Food and Drug Safety and Innovation Act, 2012 that made MDPV and all synthetic cathinones Schedule I drugs under the Controlled Substances Act (1970). While some suggest that regulation may fail to decrease harms or may actually increase harms due to potential users turning to black market providers who may use adulterated products (McElrath and O'Neill 2011), it is too early to assess the efficacy of this regulation.

4.2.5   *Lessons from Bath Salts and the Future*

One of the most interesting aspects of bath salts' emergence was the speed of the spread of information, use, and regulation. Within 2 years of its first regular reported use in a country, it caught the public's attention and was regulated. This is very much unlike salvia, which for several years has remained in federal limbo being labeled a "drug of concern," and has remained unscheduled. While its strong effects created great pressure for immediate action, one must question whether the current scheduling system and bath salts' placement in Schedule I could prevent or delay the discovery of therapeutic uses for chemicals in this category.

The use of the term bath salts to represent an array of psychoactive chemicals is itself interesting and affects both policy and research. The term originates from marketing and labeling practices shared by multiple drugs in the same general category. Whereas European clinicians and law enforcement should connect the term to mephedrone, their US equivalents should believe it to primarily represent MDPV. This distinction may be of minimal importance due to the drugs sharing many pharmacological similarities, but this may not always be the case for drugs grouped by marketing practices. The bath salts term is derived from a marketing strategy designed to circumvent the law. Future successful attempts at bypassing regulation by appearing as some other legitimate product will likely be mirrored by other novel drug producers using the same label. If the drug effects are distinct (e.g., a stimulant and a cannabinoid), confusion with deadly repercussions may arise among users, law enforcement officials, and clinicians.

Once again, the media response to an emerging drug was sensationalistic and focused only on cases with horrific outcomes. In this case, coverage promoted regulation that was likely beneficial due to the nature of the drugs' effect. However, the media could better serve the population in the future by producing accurate and non-biased reports. Future drugs with limited potential for harm may be inappropriately vilified if the pattern seen for salvia and bath salts continues. Particular insight should be derived from the Rudy Eugene and Jett McBride cases; not all bizarre and horrific behavior can be attributed to drug use. Mental health issues may be responsible for some acts, and it is therefore best to avoid linking a drug to an event until toxicology reports confirm the presence of that drug or its metabolites. Even further, use of the drug does not necessarily indicate the drug is responsible for the act. The behavior of an individual with mental health issues who uses a drug may be more the result of those issues (which may have also influenced their drug use) as opposed to the drug itself.

Finally, bath salt use presented a particular challenge for clinicians due to its rapid emergence. Given that only a limited number of case studies had explored the effects and reported appropriate treatment for someone suffering from the effects of bath salts, there was a clear lack of training among clinicians and those in public health as the number of users began to grow (Simonato et al. 2013). Since they are not regularly detected in drug screens, clinicians may be unaware that they are dealing with a patient under the influence of synthetic bath salts (Kyle et al. 2011).

Additionally, as manufacturers change the psychoactive compounds in emerging drugs to stay one step ahead of the law, they are also staying a step ahead of clinicians. The new products tweaked to avoid regulatory control may not respond to the same therapy or be as easily identified. It may take years to create tests, evaluate cases, and develop best practices by which time manufacturers will likely have switched to new formulations to skirt the law.

4.3 Case Study 3: Bromo-DragonFly, a Powerful Hallucinogen

While emerging drugs like salvia, bath salts, and synthetic cannabinoids appear to dominate media coverage, numerous other psychoactive substances have reached drug-using populations in the last several years. In some instances, the term "research chemicals" is used since the drugs may be involved in legitimate research and purchased from legitimate chemical providers. In other instances, it may be used since manufacturers label it a "research supply" to avoid regulation. One research chemical in the former category that has yet to attract mass attention is a phenethylamine called Bromo-DragonFly. This benzodifuran phenethylamine analogue (Dargan and Wood 2010) owes its name to the diagram of its chemical structure resembling a fly's body and is also referred to as spamfly, placid, and BDF.

Bromo-DragonFly was first synthesized as part of a project at Purdue University in the 1990s and appears to have transitioned to recreation use shortly after the turn of the century. At present, there are no solid assessments of its prevalence among drug users, but records of fatalities (Andreasen et al. 2009; Nielsen et al. 2010), seizures of the product (EMCDDA 2012), and Internet forums suggest that use extends beyond a handful of cases. Bromo-DragonFly is typically produced as a white or pinkish powder, but is sometimes transformed and marketed as tablets, liquid, or in blotter paper to recreational users (Dargan and Wood 2010). Coppola and Mondola (2012) suggest that the most common form of recreational use involves impregnated paper, but that insufflation, ingestion, and intravenous injection also occur.

Bromo-DragonFly's effects can most easily be compared to LSD. It is a quite potent hallucinogen with effects that can last over 24 h (Corazza et al. 2011). Users have reported that it causes euphoria, hallucinations, distorted time and space perceptions, brighter colors, sexual enhancement, diarrhea, headache, nausea, confusion, and muscle spasms (Coppola and Mondola 2012). More problematic effects have also been noted such as seizures, liver failure, renal failure, hyperpyrexia, ischemia, and death (Andreasen et al. 2009; Wood et al. 2009; Personne and Hulten 2008; Thorlacius et al. 2008). Bromo-DragonFly use seems to be limited to avid drug users, and they may use the substance in conjunction with a diverse array of other psychoactive substances (Coppola and Mondola 2012b).

Even avid drug users experience flashbacks and have claimed that the drug is too intense, too powerful, and too long-lasting (Corazza et al. 2011). Given their hesitance to promote Bromo-DragonFly to the same degree as other drugs discussed in online forums, it is questionable as to whether use will grow among drug users in the future. LSD, the drug's traditional analogue, has become less popular in recent years partially because its long action does not mesh with the demands of an increasingly interconnected modern society. With Bromo-DragonFly's effects lasting even longer than LSD's, the drug may not ever garner significant interest from casual drug users. As such, the "shadow industry" may not view the drug as being as potentially profitable as the shorter acting and more reinforcing cathinones and cannabinoids. Their market assessment may have led them to decline to invest in the production and advertisement of the product. While it may be that a negative financial assessment of the potential market prevented expenditures on Bromo-DragonFly marketing, and thus limited information reaching consumers, the lack of production could also indicate an ethical decision by producers of "legal highs." They may have chosen to withhold a product that was too potent, too dangerous, or too unpredictable. While we view this hypothesis skeptically given the inherent dangers and mass production of synthetic cathinones, it is nonetheless appropriate to question whether some form of ethics affects decision making within the "shadow industry." Regardless, it seems that there are relatively few producers and retailers of the drug (excluding those legitimate research companies only selling it in large laboratory quantities at prices well beyond the reach of individual users). Anecdotal evidence suggests that Bromo-DragonFly is far more challenging to acquire than other emerging synthetics; rather than finding it in the local "head shop," users have had to actively seek the drug to obtain it and may lack the proper lab credentials or financial means.

Given that recreational use initiated over a decade ago and has yet to become an expansive problem, Bromo-DragonFly may never be more than a chemical that a select group of avid drug users experiment with. This, however, does not imply that regulation is completely unwarranted. Only a handful of countries (e.g., Denmark, Sweden, Norway, Australia, and Romania), Oklahoma, where a young child died as a result of accidentally consuming the compound, and a few other states have expressly regulated Bromo-DragonFly (Corazza et al. 2011). Many countries such as the USA and the UK have regulations that prevent possession or use of analogues of regulated substances, but it remains to be seen whether Bromo-DragonFly is chemically similar enough to those drugs to qualify as an analogue, and it remains difficult to prosecute cases in which substances are not outright-banned. Regardless, a full ban of the substance seems imprudent given its utility in research and the security demands of working with a scheduled substance. Therefore and in light of the apparent limited recreational use, it appears that at this time an alternative approach such as product registration may be more sensible.

Bromo-DragonFly demonstrates a few insights into the novel drug phenomenon. First, unlike synthetic cannabinoids, bath salts, salvia, and other high profile novel drugs emerging around the same time, Bromo-DragonFly has never truly been a focus of popular media outlets. Other than an incident in Oklahoma that was mistakenly attributed to another drug in early reports (News9.com 2011) and a segment on "The Dr. Oz Show" (Lee 2011), the drug is largely absent from public discussion. While it could be hypothesized that the lack of media coverage is a reason use never reached quantifiable proportions, it is more likely that the undesirable extended effects deterred individuals from experimenting which, in turn, decreased the likelihood that the drug would catch the media's attention. Second, Bromo-DragonFly as a recreational drug remains underresearched despite a decade of use. Most of our understanding of the drug's recreational effects comes from the handful of cases that required medical attention or led to death. Clinicians that do deal with Bromo-DragonFly overdoses are vastly undertrained. Since there is so much unknown about Bromo-DragonFly in the recreational context, we cannot be certain that use will not escalate beyond its present scope. As such, we may not be prepared for the challenges of the future. It seems prudent to investigate emerging psychoactive substances when they first begin to reach potential drug users because we cannot be certain whether use will become relatively common as was the case for synthetic cannabinoids or remain limited as it appears was the case for the first decade of Bromo-DragonFly's recreational history.

References

ABC News. (2011). 'Imitation cocaine' killed Florida man, say authorities. *ABC News.* http://abcnews.go.com/Blotter/bath-salts-killed-florida-manauthorities/story?id=13746152. Accessed 27 Nov 2013.

Adebamiro, A., & Perazella, M. A. (2012). Recurrent acute kidney injury following bath salts intoxication. *American Journal of Kidney Diseases: The Official Journal of the National Kidney Foundation, 59*(2), 273–275.

Andreasen, M. A., Telving, R., Birkler, R. I., Schumacher, B., & Johannsen, M. (2009) A fatal poisoning involving Bromo-Dragonfly. *Forensic Science International, 183,* 91–96.

Antonowicz, J. L., Metzger, A. K., & Ramanujam, S. L. (2011). Paranoid psychosis induced by consumption of methylenedioxypyrovalerone: Two cases. *General Hospital Psychiatry, 33*(6), 640.

Appel, J., & Kim-Appel, D. (2007). The rise of a new psychoactive agent: *Salvia divinorum. International Journal of Mental Health and Addiction, 5*(3), 248–253.

Author not identified. (2011). Man threatened surgery on self, possibly high on 'bath salts.' *abc24.com.* http://www.abc24.com/news/local/story/Man-Threatened-Surgery-on-Self-Possibly-High-on/J7h5ue9Zh0yXKzk3d3hygg.cspx.

Author not identified. (2012). Bath salts: The synthetic scare. Public health and law authorities are sounding an alarm about new drugs. *The Economist.*

Baggott, M. J., Erowid, E., Erowid, F., & Mendelson, J. E. (2004). Use of *Salvia divinorum,* an unscheduled hallucinogenic plant: A web-based survey of 500 users. *Clinical Pharmacology and Therapeutics St Louis-, 75,* 72.

Baumann, M. H., Partilla, J. S., Lehner, K. R., Thorndike, E. B., Hoffman, A. F., Holy, M., Schindler, C. W., et al. (2012). Powerful cocaine-like actions of 3, 4-methylenedioxypyrovalerone (MDPV), a principal constituent of psychoactive 'bath salts' products. *Neuropsychopharmacology, 28,* 552–562.

Brandt, S. D., Freeman, S., Sumnall, H. R., Measham, F., & Cole, J. (2011). Analysis of NRG 'legal highs' in the U.K.: Identification and formation of novel cathinones. *Drug Testing and Analysis, 3*(9), 569–575.

Bücheler, R., Gleiter, C. H., Schwoerer, P., & Gaertner, I. (2005). Use of nonprohibited hallucinogenic plants: Increasing relevance for public health? A case report and literature review on the consumption of Salvia divinorum (Diviner's Sage). *Pharmacopsychiatry, 38*(1), 1–5.

Carhart-Harris, R. L., King, L. A., & Nutt, D. J. (2011). A web-based survey on mephedrone. *Drug and Alcohol Dependence, 118*(1), 19–22.

Chandra, A., & Cupps, S. (2002). E-regulation and internet pharmacies: Issues and dilemmas. *Clinical Research and Regulatory Affairs, 19*(1), 67–81.

Coppola, M. M., & Mondola, R. R. (2011). Synthetic cathinones: Chemistry, pharmacology and toxicology of a new class of designer drugs of abuse marketed as "bath salts" or "plant food". *Toxicology Letters, 211*(2), 144–149.

Coppola, M., & Mondola, R. (2012). Bromo-DragonFly: Chemistry, pharmacology and toxicology of a benzodifuran derivative producing LSD-like effects. *Journal of Addiction Research and Therapy, 3*(133), 2.

Corazza, O., Schifano, F., Farre, M., Deluca, P., Davey, Z., Drummond, C., Torrens, M., Scherbaum, N., et al. (2011). Designer drugs on the Internet: A phenomenon out-of-control? The emergence of hallucinogenic drug Bromo-Dragonfly. *Current Clinical Pharmacology, 6*(2), 125–129.

Cross, J. (2012, May 30). Despite ban, Arizona use of bath salts runs rampant. *KTAR, The Voice of Arizona*. http://ktar.com/63/1550886/Arizona-Voices. Accessed 27 Nov 2013.

Dahl, J. (2012, May 30). Bath salts, drug alleged "face-chewer" Rudy Eugene may have been on, plague police and doctors. *CBSnews*. http://www.cbsnews.com. Accessed 27 Nov 2013.

Dargan, P., & Wood, D. M. (2010). Technical profile of bromo-dragonfly. European Monitoring centre for Drugs and Drug Addiction.

Dargan, P. I., Albert, S., & Wood, D.M. (2010). Mephedrone use and associated adverse effects in school and college/university students before the U.K. legislation change. *QJM, 103*, 875–879.

Dennehy, C. E., Tsourounis, C., & Miller, A. E. (2005). Evaluation of herbal dietary supplements marketed on the internet for recreational use. *The Annals of Pharmacotherapy, 39*(10), 1634–1639.

Drug Enforcement Administration (DEA) (2013). 3,4-Methylenedioxypyrovalerone (MDPV). (Street names: "bath salts," Ivory Wave," "plant fertilizer," "Vanilla Sky," "Energy-1"). *Drug & Chemical Evaluation Section*. 1.

Dybdal-Hargreaves, N. F., Holder, N. D., Ottoson, P. E., Sweeney, M. D., & Williams, T. (2013). Mephedrone: Public health risk, mechanisms of action, and behavioral effects. *European Journal of Pharmacology, 714*, 32–40.

Erickson, T. (2011, April 13). "Bath Salt" abuse hits epidemic proportions. *Emergency Physicians Monthly*. http://www.epmonthly.com/. Accessed 27 Nov 2013.

European Monitoring Centre for Drugs and Drug Abuse (EMCDDA) (2012). Statistical bulletin 2012 Other substances seized, 2004–2010. http://www.emcdda.europa.eu/stats12/szrtab21a. Accessed 27 Nov 2013.

Fass, J. A., Fass, A. D., & Garcia, A. S. (2012). Synthetic cathinones (bath salts): Legal status and patterns of abuse. *The Annals of Pharmacotherapy, 46*(3), 436–41.

Freeman, T. P., Morgan, C. J., Vaughn-Jones, J., Hussain, N., Karimi, K., & Curran, H.V. (2012). Cognitive and subjective effects of mephedrone and factors influencing use of a 'new legal high'. *Addiction, 107*, 792–800.

Giroud, C., Felber, F., Augsburger, M., Horisberger, B., Rivier, L., & Mangin, P. (2000). *Salvia divinorum*: An hallucinogenic mint which might become a new recreational drug in Switzerland. *Forensic Science International, 112*(2), 143–150.

González, D., Riba, J., Bouso, J. C., Gómez-Jarabo, G., & Barbanoj, M. J. (2006). Pattern of use and subjective effects of *Salvia divinorum* among recreational users. *Drug and Alcohol Dependence, 85*(2), 157–162.

Griffin, O. H., III., Miller, B. L., & Khey, D. N. 2008. Legally high? Legal considerations of Salvia divinorum. *Journal of Psychoactive Drugs, 40*, 183–191.

Gustavsson, D., & Escher, C. (2009). Mephedrone—Internet drug which seems to have come and stay. Fatal cases in Sweden have drawn attention to previously unknown substances. *Lakartidningen, 106*, 2769–2777.

Hiaasesn, S., & Green, N., (2012). No bath salts detected: Causeway attacker Rudy Eugene had only pot in his system, medical examiner reports. *The Miami Herald*. http://www.miamiherald.com/. Accessed 27 Nov 2013.

Hoover, V., Marlowe, D. B., Patapis, N. S., Festinger, D. S., & Forman, R. F. (2008). Internet access to Salvia divinorum: Implications for policy, prevention, and treatment. *Journal of Substance Abuse Treatment, 35*(1), 22–27.

Johnson, G. (2011, April 22). Bath salt drugs found on man in murder-suicide. *The Huffington Post.* http://www.huffingtonpost.com/. Accessed 27 Nov 2013.

Johnston, L. D., O'Malley, P. M., Bachman, J. G., & Schulenberg, J. E. (2013). *Monitoring the Future national results on adolescent drug use: Overview of key findings, 2012.* Ann Arbor: Institute for Social Research, The University of Michigan, p. 83.

Karila, L., & Reynaud, M. (2011). GHB and synthetic cathinones: Clinical effects and potential consequences. *Drug Testing and Analysis, 9,* 552–559.

Khan, S., Shaheen, F., Sarwar, H., Molina, J., & Mushtaq, S. (2013). "Bath salts"-induced psychosis in a young woman. *Primary Care Companion to the Journal of Clinical Psychiatry, 15,* 1.

Khey, D. N., Miller, B. L., & Griffin, O. H. (2008). *Salvia divinorum* use among a college student sample. *Journal of Drug Education, 38*(3), 297–306.

Kriikku, P., Wilhelm, L., Schwarz, O., & Rintatalo, J. (2011). New designer drug of abuse: 3,4-methylenedioxypyrovalerone (MDPV). Findings from apprehended drivers in Finland. *Forensic Science International, 210,* 195–200.

Kyle, P. B., Iverson, R. B., Gajagowni, R. G., & Spencer, L. (2011). Illicit bath salts: Not for bathing. *Journal of the Mississippi State Medical Association, 52*(12), 375.

Lange, J. E., Daniel, J., Homer, K., Reed, M. B., & Clapp, J. D. (2010). *Salvia divinorum*: Effects and use among YouTube users. *Drug and Alcohol Dependence, 108,* 138–140.

Lee, J. (2011). Dragonfly: What this deadly new drug means for your family. *The Dr. Oz Show.* http://www.doctoroz.com/videos/dragonfly-what-deadly-new-drug-means-your-family. Accessed 27 Nov 2013.

Lehner, K. R., & Baumann, M. H. (2013). Psychoactive 'Bath Salts': compounds, mechanisms, and toxicities. *Neuropsychopharmacology, 38*(1), 243–244.

McElrath, K., & O'Neill, C. (2011) Experiences with mephedrone pre- and post-legislative controls: Perceptions of safety and sources of supply. *International Journal of Drug Policy, 22*(2), 120–127.

McNamara, S., Stokes, S., & Coleman, N. (2010) Head shop compound abuse amongst attendees of the Drug Treatment Centre Board. *Internal Medicine Journal, 103,* 134–137.

Meyer, M. R., Wilhelm, J., Peters, F. T., & Maurer, H. H. (2010). Beta-keto amphetamines: Studies on the metabolism of the designer drug mephedrone and toxicological detection of mephedrone, butylone, and methylone in urine using gas chromatography-mass spectrometry. *Analytical and Bioanalytical Chemistry, 397*(3), 1225–1233.

Murray, B. L., Murphy, C. M., & Beuhler, M. C. (2012). Death following recreational use of designer drug "bath salts" containing 3, 4-Methylenedioxypyrovalerone (MDPV). *Journal of Medical Toxicology: Official Journal of the American College of Medical Toxicology, 8*(1), 69–75.

Nelson, S. (2012). Pamela McCarthy, naked 'bath salts' mother who choked son, 3, dies after being tasered by police. *Huffington Post UK.* http://www.huffingtonpost.co.uk/. Accessed 27 Nov 2013.

News9.com. (2011). Second victim dies after taking designer drug in Konawa. http://www.newson6. com/story/14641463/second-victim-dies-after-taking-designer-drug-in-konawa. Accessed 27 Nov 2013.

Nielsen, V. T., Høgberg, L. C., & Behrens, J. K. (2010). Bromo-Dragonfly poisoning of 18-year-old male. *Ugeskrift for laeger, 172*(19), 1461.

Pavarin, R. M. (2006). Substance use and related problems: A study on the abuse of recreational and not recreational drugs in Northern Italy. *Annali Dell'istituto Superiore Di Sanitá, 42*(4), 477–484.

Penders, T. M., & Gestring, R. (2011). Hallucinatory delirium following use of MDPV: "Bath Salts". *General Hospital Psychiatry, 33*(5), 525–526.

Personne, M., & Hulten, P. (2008) Bromo-Dragonfly a life threatening designer drug. *Clinical Toxicology, 46,* 379–380.

Porrovecchio, A. (2011). Bath salts that were never meant for a tub. *American College of Physicians.* http://www.acphospitalist.org/archives/2011/11/perspectives.htm. Accessed 27 Nov 2013.

Prisinzano, T. E. (2005). Psychopharmacology of the hallucinogenic sage *Salvia divinorum*. *Life Sciences, 78*(5), 527–531.

Prosser, L. M., Nelson, L. S. (2012). The toxicology of bath salts: A review of synthetic cathinones. *Journal of Medical Toxicology, 8,* 33–42.

Roff, A. N., (2012). Bath salts: A 'scary' and growing epidemic. *Utica Observer Dispatch.* http://www.uticaod.com/. Accessed 27 Nov 2013.

Rome, J. (eotl3). (2013). Jim Rome has hilarious take on Kai the Homeless Hatchet Man (Video file). http://www.youtube.com/watch?v=ZzkBlleZmkM. Accessed 27 Nov 2013.

Ross, E. A., Watson, M., & Goldberger, B. (2011) "Bath salts" intoxication. *New England Journal of Medicine, 365*(10), 967–968.

Schifano, F., Fergus, S., Stair, J. L., Corazza, O., Albanese, A., Corkery, J., Ghodse, A. H., & Haugen, L. S. Y. (2011). Mephedrone (4-methylmethcathinone; 'Meow meow'): Chemical, pharmacological and clinical issues. *Psychopharmacology, 214*(3), 593–602.

Sheridan, M. (2011, May 5). Mark Thompson, found in women's lingerie standing over dead goat, was high on 'bath salts.' *New York Daily News.* http://www.nydailynews.com. Accessed 27 Nov 2013.

Simonato, P., Corazza, O., Santonastaso, P., Corkery, J., Deluca, P., Davey, Z., Schifano, F., et al. (2013). Novel psychoactive substances as a novel challenge for health professionals: results from an Italian survey. *Human Psychopharmacology: Clinical and Experimental, 28*(4), 324–331.

Spiller, H. A., Ryan, M. L., Weston, R. G., & Jansen, J. (2011, January 1). Clinical experience with and analytical confirmation of "bath salts" and "legal highs" (synthetic cathinones) in the United States. *Clinical Toxicology, 49*(6), 499–505.

Spring, T. (2009). 'Salvia killed my son,' Says Mother. *PCWorld.* http://abcnews.go.com/Technology/PCWorld/story?id=6782912. Accessed 27 Nov 2013.

Stogner, J. M., & Miller, B. L. (2013). Investigating the 'bath salt' panic: The rarity of synthetic cathinone use among students in the United States. *Drug and alcohol review, 32*(5), 545–549.

Stogner, J., Khey, D. N., Griffin, O. H., Miller, B. L., & Boman, J. H. (2012). Regulating a novel drug: an evaluation of changes in use of *Salvia divinorum* in the first year of Florida's ban. *The International Journal on Drug Policy, 23*(6), 512–21.

Streur, W. J., Hurlburt, W. B., McLaughlin, J., & Castrodale, L. (Eds.). (2011). Psychoactive "bath salts" toxicity in Alaska-a case series, Bulletin. *State of Alaska Epidemiology, 27,* 1.

Substance Abuse and Mental Health Services Administration (SAMHSA). (2007). Results from the 2006 National Survey on Drug Use and Health: National Findings. *NSDUH Series H-32, DHHS Publication No. SMA,* 07-4293.

Substance Abuse and Mental Health Services Administration (SAMHSA) (2012). Results from the 2011 National Survey on Drug Use and Health: Summary of National Findings and Detailed Tables. http://www.samhsa.gov/data/NSDUH/2011SummNatFindDetTables/Index.aspx.

Thorlacius, K., Borna C., & Personne, M. (2008) Bromo-dragon fly-life-threatening drug. Can cause tissue necrosis as demonstrated by the first described case. *Lakartidningen, 105,* 1199–1200.

Wasson, R. G. (1962). A new Mexican psychotropic drug from the mint family. *Botanical Museum Leaflets Harvard University, 20*(3), 77–84.

Westphal, F., Junge, T., Rosner, P., Sonnichsen, F., & Schuster, F. (2009). Mass and NMR spectroscopic characterization of 3,4-methylenedioxypyrovalerone: A designer drug with @a-pyrrolidinophenone structure. *Forensic Science International, 190,* 1–8.

Winder, G. S., Stern, N., & Hosanagar, A. (2013). Are "Bath Salts" the next generation of stimulant abuse?. *Journal of Substance Abuse Treatment, 44*(1), 42–45.

Winstock, A., Mitcheson, L., & Marsden, J. (2010). Mephedrone: Still available and twice the price. *Lancet, 376*(9752), 1537.

Winstock, A. R., Mitcheson, L. R., Deluca, P., Davey, Z., Corazza, O., & Schifano, F. (2011). Mephedrone, new kid for the chop? *Addiction, 106*(1), 154–161.

Wood, D. M., Looker, J. J., Shaikh, L., Button, J., & Puchnarewicz, M., et al. (2009) Delayed onset of seizures and toxicity associated with recreational use of Bromo-Dragonfly. *Journal of Medical Toxicology, 5,* 226–229.

Wright M. J., Jr., Vandewater, S. A., Angrish, D., Dickerson, T. J., & Taffe, M. A. (2012). Mephedrone (4-methylmethcathinone) and d-methamphetamine improve visuospatial associative memory, but not spatial working memory, in rhesus macaques. *British Journal of Pharmacology, 167*(6), 1342–1352.

Zawilska, J. B., & Wojcieszak, J. (2013). *Salvia divinorum*: From Mazatec medicinal and hallucinogenic plant to emerging recreational drug. *Human Psychopharmacology: Clinical and Experimental, 28*(5), 403–412.

Chapter 5
What Is Being Done About Emerging Drugs?

In recent years, at both the state and federal level (even a few rare local ordinances) have addressed a perceived threat in several American communities in the past decade. However, there does not appear to be any consistency on how these substances are regulated nor on who should be primarily responsible for their oversight. The divergence between state and federal drug laws regarding emerging drugs is particularly noteworthy as inconsistent policies appear to be increasingly common. Along with the legal mechanisms to regulate emerging drugs, many challenges exist in the enforcement and detection of these substances. At this time, only a few local jurisdictions appear to be taking a proactive enforcement role at any level. Federal regulators have been more active in focusing on cases dealing with large volumes of product, but rarely center efforts on end users. This chapter outlines the mechanisms in which new drugs are regulated and how these policies are enforced. It also explores the impact of these regulations and their enforcement on usage.

5.1 The Controlled Substances Act

Intoxicants have been regulated in diverse ways throughout the history of USA. Whether by including an amendment to the constitution, developing provisions that amend tax law, enacting local, state, or federal laws, the country has creatively tried to subdue the use of psychoactive substances for well over a century. Partially due to this complexity and years of inconsistency, the federal government began regulating substances under a unified method in 1970. The Controlled Substances Act (CSA) placed near complete control of psychoactive substances in the hands of the federal government. This legislation outlined a scheduling framework based on medical use and safety profile, or "abuse liability," of psychoactive substances. Put simply, drugs could be categorized in one of five tiers or "schedules," each of which was linked to a certain level of regulation.

The CSA granted the Drug Enforcement Administration (DEA) the ability to schedule psychoactive substances based on these criteria. Therefore, the CSA intended to place primary responsibility for determining which substances were to be regulated and how to regulate them in the hands of the DEA. Furthermore, the CSA set

D. N. Khey et al., *Emerging Trends in Drug Use and Distribution*,
SpringerBriefs in Criminology 12, DOI 10.1007/978-3-319-03575-8_5,
© Springer International Publishing Switzerland 2014

up protocols for changes. The US Department of Health and Human Services (HHS) may submit a petition to add, delete, upgrade, or downgrade a substance within the CSA, or the DEA may initiate an investigation itself. The DEA's investigation of a substance includes gathering information from law enforcement laboratories, state and local law enforcement, regulatory agencies, and experts in order to determine if scheduling is necessary (Yeh 2012).

The CSA set up a five-tier system for classifying and regulating substances. According to the law, a Schedule I substance indicates that the drug or substance has "no currently accepted medical use in treatment in the United States," and a "high potential for abuse," thus having "a lack of accepted safety for use of the drug or other substance under medical supervision" (21 U.S.C. § 812). Lysergic acid diethylamide (LSD), marijuana, heroin, ecstasy, and peyote are examples of substances classified as Schedule I at the federal level. Schedule II indicates that the substance has a high potential for abuse (e.g., may lead to severe physical and/or psychological dependence), yet also has a currently accepted medical use in treatment in the USA. This schedule includes substances such as methamphetamine, cocaine, morphine, and hydrocodone. For Schedule III substances, the potential for abuse is less than the substances in Schedules I and II (e.g., the abuse of the substance may lead to moderate or low physical and/or psychological dependence). Ketamine, anabolic steroids, and buprenorphine are Schedule III drugs. Schedule IV substances such as pentazocine (Talwin), phenobarbital, and clonazepam (Klonopin) are considered to have a lower potential for abuse relative to Schedule III substances (e.g., the abuse may lead to limited physical and/or psychological dependence). Lastly, Schedule V substances have the lowest potential for abuse; this classification is mostly reserved for anti-diarrhea drugs, cough suppressants, and very mild analgesics (pain-relievers).

It is through this five-level system of classifying drugs and substances that the government has instituted most drug policies in the last 40 years. Schedule I substances are considered to be illicit drugs with no medical value by the federal government. Thus, their possession is banned in almost all contexts other than highly secure research studies (although federal regulation of some substances is effectively ignored at some local levels). The CSA is consistently evolving with the DEA using its scheduling powers to place emerging drugs into varying levels of regulation.

5.1.1 Emergency Scheduling Powers

In 1984, the CSA was amended by the Comprehensive Crime Control Act that allowed the attorney general to place a drug or substance into Schedule I of the CSA on a temporary basis. This emergency scheduling power was intended to avoid an "imminent hazard to public safety" (21 U.S.C. § 811) and can effectively restrict possession of a substance in less than a month. This power has since been delegated to the deputy administrator of the DEA and is used to regulate emerging drugs perceived as a potential threat. The deputy administrator (in lieu of the attorney general) must give 30 days notice to the general public and the HHS secretary prior to the ban and consider the HHS Secretary's position regarding the use of emergency scheduling.

In 2012, the Synthetic Drug Abuse Prevention Act was passed which further clarified the process for emergency or temporary scheduling (Yeh 2012). The language was altered to clarify that the attorney general (or his/her designee as identified by law—e.g., the deputy administrator) must consider for an "imminent hazard to public safety (i) the history of the drug or substance and its current pattern of abuse; (ii) the scope, duration, and significance of the drug or substance's abuse; (iii) the risk to public health; (iv) diversion of the drug or substance from legitimate channels; and (v) the drug or substance's 'clandestine importation, manufacture, or distribution'" (Yeh 2012, p. 3). Emergency scheduling is intended to be temporary and substances may only be placed in Schedule I under this provision if they have no accepted medical use in the USA. Emergency scheduling is initially for a 2-year period, but an additional year may be added if the formal scheduling process has been initiated (Yeh 2012). It has been through the emergency scheduling process that many emerging drugs were initially regulated.

The DEA began using this temporary scheduling process in 1985. While MDMA (ecstasy) was the first to make headlines, it was actually the second drug to be placed in Schedule I through the emergency scheduling powers (a short 2 months after instituting emergency scheduling powers, 3-methylfentanyl was placed in Schedule I on March 25, 1985). During the publicized hearings on how to permanently schedule MDMA, most experts recommended a Schedule III placement due to the possible medical use of MDMA in psychotherapy. Disregarding these recommendations, the drug was placed into Schedule I until in 1987 the First Circuit Court of Appeals remanded the scheduling determination temporarily removing it from Schedule I (Grinspoon vs. Drug Enforcement Administration 1987). Despite objections from the medical community, MDMA was placed back into Schedule I status after a reevaluation in 1988.

Following the ban on MDMA, several other drugs have been emergency scheduled including the psychedelic substances 2C-B (4-bromo-2,5-dimethoxyphenethylamine) and AMT (alpha-Methyltryptamine), stimulants such as BZP (Benzylpiperazine) and MDPV (Methylenedioxypyrovalerone), and synthetic cannabinoids (JWH-018 and CP 47,497). In 2004, TFMPP's (3-Trifluoro-methylphenylpiperazine) emergency scheduling expired and was not renewed. This is the only case in which a drug has been emergency scheduled and later became a legal substance. Although TFMPP is an unscheduled substance federally, several states have regulated the substance.

5.1.2   Controlled Substance Analogues

As a result of the creation of new synthetic substances that chemically resembled and had effects similar to controlled substances, the Federal Analogue Act was passed in

1986. It amended the CSA to include substances that are not controlled but are "substantially similar" structurally or pharmacologically to substances found in Schedule I or II (21 U.S.C. § 813). A "controlled substance analogue" that is intended for human consumption is treated as if it were a controlled substance in Schedule I or II.

Though the Act attempted to clarify what qualifies as a controlled substance analogue (see 21 U.S.C. § 802 definition 32), there is still a substantial amount of gray area. Within the definition, there is no description of how similar substances' chemical structures have to be in order for them to meet the criteria of being "substantially similar." The law also does not describe how comparable effects on the central nervous system have to be to be considered "substantially similar" or whether this refers to perceived psychoactive effects or more easily quantified chemical effects. These issues appear to be left for the courts to decide. At the state level, regulation has clarified that "isomers, esters, ethers, salts, or salts of isomers, esters, and ethers" of banned compounds are similarly banned (Florida House Bill 1363 2008), but no clarification exists at the federal level. This issue has led some to challenge that the policy is unconstitutionally vague and is therefore void (USA vs. Forbes, 806 F. Supp. 232 1992), but it remains intact.

The most glaring weakness of the Federal Analogue Act is its provision that excludes "any substance to the extent not intended for human consumption" (21 U.S.C. § 802). As such, only those products marketed with explicit use of human ingestion, injection, or inhalation are subject to the ban. As a means of bypassing controlled substance analogue policies, manufacturers of emerging drugs specifically market their products as "not for human consumption" though they fully intend them to be consumed by purchasers. The "not for human consumption" designation also allows products to bypass the regulations of the Federal Food and Drug Administration (FDA) which is charged with supervising the development, safety, and security of all products directly ingested or applied to the body (pharmaceuticals, foods, medical devices, cosmetics, etc.).

5.1.3   Food and Drug Administration

The vast majority of what we now consider illicit drugs has their origins as pharmaceutical products. From Bayer's marketing of heroin to the first recipe of Coca-Cola including cocaine, drugs were often originally designated as household medicines and remedies for all types of ailments. The patent-medicine industry at the turn of the twentieth century included a large number of tonics and potions with primary ingredients such as cocaine, morphine, heroin, and alcohol (Spillane 2000). Due to the large number of people experiencing adverse side effects including dependencies, the Pure Food and Drug Act of 1906 was passed prohibiting the "manufacture, sale, or transportation of adulterated or misbranded or poisonous or deleterious foods, drugs, medicines, and liquors." This legislature required patent medicines to disclose their ingredients and led to the collapse of the industry and formation of the modern pharmaceutical industry and its regulatory body.

Originally known as the Bureau of Chemistry, the US Food and Drug Administration currently regulates existing pharmaceuticals and evaluates new ones. New products must go through a rigorous testing process to ensure that they are safe enough for human consumption. A criticism of this current model is that the modern process in which to bring a new drug to market can take up to 10 years and an estimated US$ 800 million (Goozner 2004). Some of those innovating in the area of pharmacotherapy choose to circumvent the lengthy legitimate process of creating medications by labeling products as "not for human consumption." Indeed, manufacturers of emerging drugs seem to use this criticism of the FDA as a justification for their practices. For example, www.libertyherb.com clarifies on their website that the reason their products are labeled not for human consumption is "Because of this claim, botanical herbal incense is not technically classified as a food or a drug, and thus, the Herbal Incense industry can offer its products to the market directly at an affordable price to consumer market place." The website then offers information criticizing the FDA process to further legitimize their products and mislead consumers about their safety.

5.2 A Move Away from the CSA

As the CSA is the overarching framework for all US drug policy and includes guidelines for the scheduling of substances, the majority of states have developed their own scheduling processes and laws that parallel the CSA. Following the passage of the CSA, state laws generally mirrored federal laws and substances were similarly scheduled by federal and state agencies. However, the USA has a complex two-tiered system of criminal justice with potential for divergent laws and policies. The violation of federal laws is enforced by federal law enforcement and tried in federal courts whereas state laws are enforced by local police, sheriffs, and state law enforcement and tried within state courts. Because drugs are both regulated at the federal and state level, this can create a complicated situation when state and federal laws are not congruent. These unresolved legal issues of federalism are becoming more common as related to drug use.

Two relatively new phenomena have recently highlighted the potential for inconsistent federal and local drug policies to exist and are currently confusing both drug users and law enforcement. First, the hesitance of the federal government to schedule certain emerging drugs has created a situation where states are differentially banning substances. Until the last decade, the Federal government typically scheduled new substances as their abuse potential became evident, but several substances, in the absence of federal action, have been regulated only at the state level. Second, states have challenged the CSA classification of marijuana as a Schedule I substance allowing for its medical use and creating a situation in which drug control has been shifted back to the state level. This state-level medicalization (and even decriminalization) of marijuana has created a scenario where a substance that is legal to possess in the eyes of local government is illicit as far as the federal government is concerned.

These two examples, discussed in detail in the following sections, may foreshadow an impending shift in the framework of US drug policy.

5.2.1   State-Level Medicalization of Marijuana

Medical marijuana exists in a complex legal paradox in the USA. Twenty states and the District of Columbia have passed provisions to allow for the medical use of marijuana, but marijuana remains a Schedule I substance and, by definition of the federal government, it has no accepted medical use in the USA. As recently as August 2013, the White House has clarified that President Obama does not favor the rescheduling of marijuana "at this point," even following the highly publicized endorsement from CNN chief medical correspondent Dr. Sanjay Gupta (Blake 2013). On August 20th 2013, White House spokesman Josh Earnest clarified the Obama Administration's position, "while the prosecution of drug trafficking remains an important priority, the president and the administration believe that targeting individual marijuana users, especially those with serious illnesses and their caregivers, is not the best allocation of federal law enforcement resources" (Johnson and Chebium 2013).

Although the DEA may not be targeting individual users in states that have passed medical marijuana provisions, the current administration has spent nearly US$ 300 million on medical marijuana intervention through lawsuits, indictments, and penalties. The Internal Revenue Service also appears to be targeting and attacking medical marijuana dispensaries and the medical marijuana industry (Americans for Safe Access 2013). This issue is likely to soon become one that President Obama and the federal government cannot ignore or brush aside. The recent "legalization" of marijuana in Colorado and Washington further complicates the situation and calls for an official decision by federal agencies. With the first marijuana retail stores opening in Colorado as soon as 2014, even more tension may develop between state and federal drug policies (Fig. 5.1).

5.2.2   Salvia divinorum, Kratom, and other State Level Bans

Several states have also taken the initiative to ban substances prior to action by the federal government. One of the earliest modern examples of this is in the banning of *Salvia divinorum*. A bill proposed in 2002 would have placed salvia into Schedule I of the CSA, but died in committee (Griffin et al. 2008). The DEA listed salvia as a "drug of concern," but has not used its emergency scheduling powers to regulate it nor has it completed the formal process of scheduling it. The result of the inaction by the federal government has led to various prohibitions of salvia in 34 states (Vandrey et al., 2013).

The very first law banning salvia in the USA was a municipal law passed in the small town of Saint Peters, Missouri. This law was a response to accounts of

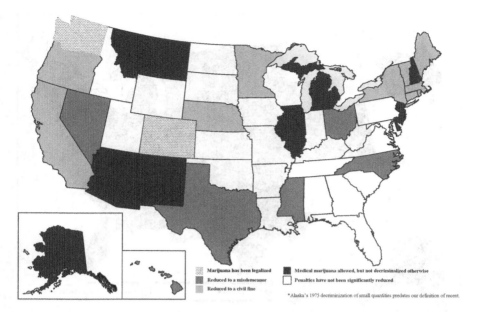

Fig. 5.1 Recent US marijuana policy changes

teenagers using salvia and restricted the sale to only those over the age of 18 (Griffin et al. 2008). Louisiana became the first state to ban the production, manufacture, and distribution of salvia in 2005. The Louisiana law prohibits several plants with hallucinogenic properties and specifically mentions 41 plants by name including *S. divinorum*. Later in 2005, Missouri placed *S. divinorum* and the active compound salvinorin A into Schedule I of the Missouri Controlled Substance Act (Stogner et al. 2012). The substantial media coverage following the 2006 suicide of a Delaware teenager with a history of salvia use prompted several states to take action to regulate salvia. Regulations have taken several forms including age restriction, scheduling the substance, or enacting a specific law (Stogner et al. 2012).

A number of states have added *S. divinorum* and/or the active ingredient salvinorin A to their state CSA including: Delaware (2006), Oklahoma (2006), North Dakota (2007), Florida (2008), Illinois (2008), Kansas (2008), Mississippi (2008), Virginia (2008), Hawaii (2009), Nebraska (2009), Ohio (2009), South Dakota (2009), Alabama (2010), Georgia (2010), Kentucky (2010), Michigan (2010), Minnesota (2010), Connecticut (2011), Indiana (2011), Iowa (2011), Pennsylvania (2011), Wyoming (2011), Arkansas (2012), and Colorado (2012). Other states chose to enact separate legislation for salvia in a manner similar to Louisiana's salvia ban. In 2006, Tennessee prohibited the possession of salvinorin A. In 2009, North Carolina prohibited both *S. divinorum* and salvinorin A. A 2010 law in West Virginia only prohibits "processed" salvia. In 2010, Wisconsin prohibited the manufacture, distribution,

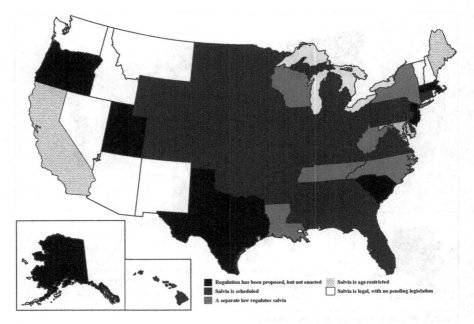

Fig. 5.2 Legal status of salvia regulation in the USA

or delivering of salvinorin A but not possession (Stogner et al. 2012). In 2012, New York prohibited only the sale of *S. divinorum* but not possession (Fig. 5.2).

Rather than banning it completely, several states have placed age restrictions on salvia. In 2007, Maine passed a law prohibiting anyone under the age of 18 from possessing salvia. California passed a law in 2009 prohibiting the sale of *S. divinorum* or salvinorin A to minors, but did not ban possession. In 2010, Maryland passed a law prohibiting the possession of *S. divinorum* or salvinorin A to anyone under the age of 21.

Of the 16 states that have not passed regulations restricting salvia, seven of the states have proposed regulations on salvia that have either failed to pass or died in committee (Alaska, Massachusetts, New Jersey, Oregon, South Carolina, Texas, and Utah). Currently, legislation to regulate salvia has not been introduced in Arizona, Idaho, Montana, Nevada, New Hampshire, New Mexico, Rhode Island, Vermont, or Washington. Despite two-thirds of American states regulating salvia, the federal government remains on the sideline in managing regulation of the drug.

Kratom (*Mitragyna speciosa*) is another example of a substance that has been subject to statewide bans. Kratom is a plant that natively grows in Thailand and Malaysia and has been used for thousands of years for its sedative properties. The DEA has listed kratom on its list of "drugs and chemicals of concern," but has not utilized its scheduling powers. One state has banned kratom; in 2012, Indiana House Bill 1196 added the two active alkaloids of kratom (mitragynine and 7-hydroxymitragynine) to Schedule I of the state CSA. Interestingly, the bill included the active ingredients of kratom as a "synthetic drug" along with a long list of synthetic cannabinoids and stimulants, yet we note that kratom products contain the plant product and are not typically considered "synthetic substances." Further confusion over this issue is evident when an Iowa bill was proposed listing *Mitragyna speciosa* as a synthetic cannabinoid (Iowa Senate Bill 2341 2012). The only other state that has regulated kratom is Louisiana, which passed a law prohibiting the distribution of *M. speciosa* to minors. Several other states have considered various forms of regulations on kratom (Arizona, Hawaii, Iowa, Massachusetts, Tennessee, Vermont, and Virginia).

5.3   Synthetic Cannabinoids, Bath Salts, and the Synthetic Drug Abuse Prevention Act of 2012

The federal government has acted and acted fairly quickly on two emerging substances. Both synthetic cannabinoids and "bath salt" products, containing synthetic cathinones and/or MDPV, were marketed as "not for human consumption" in order to avoid being considered an illicit analogue. Similar to salvia, state level bans on these substances started to emerge; but soon following these bans, the DEA used the emergency scheduling powers under the CSA to prohibit the sale and possession of these products. One of the challenges of regulating synthetic legal intoxicating drugs (SLIDs) is that there is often a large group of compounds that produce similar effects and each marketed product may be chemically unique (see Jerry et al. 2012). When a compound is banned, manufacturers often simply claim to have replaced that compound with others and at other times attempt to bypass regulations by replacing that specific compound in their formula with other synthetic compounds that have similar effects (Jerry et al. 2012). This creates a situation in which a cat and mouse game is often played where new products similar to the banned ones replace the old (and illegal) substances (often even under the same brand name), but contain chemical compounds different than those regulated.

Starting around 2008, the US Military Services passed several policies banning the use of synthetic cannabinoids among service members (Vardakou et al. 2010). Kansas was the first state to ban the use of synthetic cannabinoids in March 2010 and several other states passed legislation banning synthetic cannabinoid compounds prior to federal action (Vardakou et al. 2010). There is a wide variety of synthetic cannabinoids that can be applied to herbal mixtures to create psychoactive products that mimic the effects of cannabis, and this diversity presents a challenge for lawmakers. On March 1, 2011 the DEA placed the five most common chemicals in the K2 and Spice brands (JWH-018, JWH-073, JWH-200, CP-47 497, and CP-47 497 C8 homologue) into Schedule I of the CSA on an emergency basis. Following the ban of some psychoactive compounds, new formulations were rotated onto the market. On July 9, 2012 the Synthetic Drug Abuse Prevention portion of the Food and Drug Safety and Innovation Act was signed into law by the president placing "any substance that is a cannabinoid receptor type 1 (CB1 receptor) agonist" into Schedule I (Food and Drug Safety and Innovation Act 2012). This act specifically named all known synthetic cannabinoids and allows for newly discovered compounds to be placed into Schedule I.

In early 2011, several states began passing laws banning bath salt products, and by September 2011, the federal government placed a 1-year ban on the sale and possession of any substance containing MDPV, mephedrone, or methylone. This temporary ban was issued in order for the DEA to collect data and evaluate if these substances should be permanently included as Schedule I substances under the CSA. As has been the case for most drugs that have been emergency scheduled, the ban soon became permanent. In the permanent ban, the USA legislated control over the entire category rather than specific compounds. The Synthetic Drug Abuse Prevention Act of 2012 placed MDPV and all synthetic cathinones into Schedule I of the CSA.

5.4 International Regulations of Emerging Drugs

A large number of countries have also placed regulations on emerging substances. For example, a number of countries have banned salvia including Australia, Belgium, Canada, Chile, Croatia, Czech Republic, Denmark, Finland, Germany, Ireland, Italy, Latvia, Lithuania, New Zealand, Poland, Romania, Russia, Spain, Sweden, and the UK. However, kratom has only been banned in a handful of countries including Australia, Malaysia, Myanmar, and Thailand. A large number of European countries have regulated synthetic cannabinoids (Castellanos et al. 2011; Vardakou et al. 2010) along with Australia, Canada, Chile, Japan, New Zealand, South Korea, and the United Arab Emirates. Bath salt products have been banned in Australia, Canada, Denmark, Finland, Sweden, and the UK.

Some emerging drugs have not made their way to the USA in widespread use, but have become popular in other contexts. Due to the complexity of international drug regulation and the fad aspect of drug use, particularly when it comes to emerging substances, some substances have emerged as drugs of concern in geographically isolated places. For instance, although bath salts products in the USA largely consisted of MDPV, prior to these products becoming available in the USA, mephedrone-based products became popular and were regulated in the UK. Similarly, TFMPP (3-Trifluoromethylphenylpiperazine) became popular and was subsequently banned in New Zealand, but never became popular in the USA and was the first drug to have its emergency scheduling expire without being permanently added to the CSA.

5.5 Law Enforcement and Interdiction

Emerging drugs present a large number of challenges to law enforcement. One of the greatest of these challenges, given the ever-changing nature of emerging drugs, is the training of law enforcement personnel on how to recognize these substances and

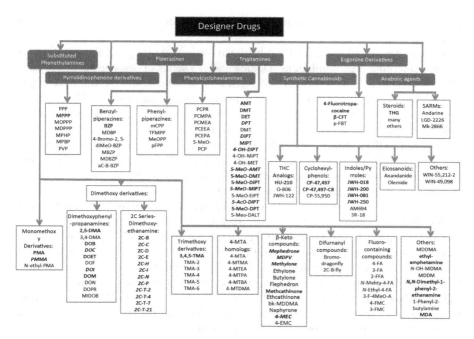

Fig. 5.3 A taxonomy of designer drugs. (Reproduced and adapted from Boos 2011 and Wohlfarth and Weinmann 2010).

also understanding their complex and often fluid legal status. Most police officers receive extensive training on how to identify traditional illicit drugs (marijuana, cocaine, methamphetamines, and heroin), but it has only been recently and very sporadically that training for emerging drugs have become available. DEA agents, and perhaps local and state police officers as part of a narcotics task force, may be knowledgeable about these substances, but the vast majority of local police, sheriffs, and state highway enforcement officers have not received specialized training on how to recognize and deal with emerging drugs.

To illustrate the difficulties in drug enforcement of emerging drugs, in a 2011 presentation by the Drug and Chemical Evaluation (ODE) section of the DEA Office of Diversion Control, an elaborate diagram of designer drugs outlining the various legal statuses of these substances at the time was released (Boos 2011). In this diagram, emerging substances were identified which have been controlled, may be possible isomers, and those determined to fall under the controlled substance analogue provisions of the CSA (Fig. 5.3).

This issue is further compounded given the differences from state to state, and when an officer is unaware of what substance may actually be contained in a product being sold as "herbal incense," "bath salts," or under some other form of branding. Often users, distributors, sellers, and even manufacturers are uncertain of what chemicals are contained in these products prior to laboratory testing. This creates a daunting task for law enforcement in their ability to identify and enforce the law on emerging drugs.

Despite these challenges, the DEA has been successful in large-scale operations to enforce emerging drug regulations. Domestically, a series of raids began on July 25, 2012 that resulted in the seizure of US$ 36 million in cash, almost 5 million packages of synthetic cannabinoids, and a large quantity of bath salt products (DEA 2012). The operation known as "Log Jam" resulted in the arrest of over 90 people and $ 6 million in asset forfeitures. The DEA in concert with the US Immigration Customs Enforcement (ICE), the Internal Revenue Service (IRS) Criminal Investigations, the US Postal Inspection Service, the US Customs Border Protection (CBP), the Federal Bureau of Investigations (FBI), the Food and Drug Administration's Office of Criminal Investigations, and local police agencies conducted raids in 30 different states. The main goal of these raids was to disrupt the flow of assets (including the $ 36 million in cash) used to finance the manufacture of emerging drugs.

On December 1, 2012 the DEA began "Project Synergy"—the largest international interdiction program to identify and bring to justice manufacturers and traffickers of illicit designer drugs (DEA 2013). The DEA's Special Operations Division coordinated the project along with support from the DEA Office of Diversion Control, CBP, ICE, FBI, IRS, Homeland Security Investigations (HSI), and a large number of state and local law enforcement agencies. This international investigation also involved cooperation from law enforcement agencies in Australia, Barbados, Panama, and Canada. As of July 2013, the result of this large-scale targeted effort was over 227 arrests, $ 51 million in assets seized, and 416 search warrants issued in 35 states, 49 cities, and five countries (DEA 2013). The operation was able to confiscate nearly 10,000 kg of individually packaged and ready-to-sell products containing illicit forms of synthetic drugs. This included nearly 300 kg of bath salt products containing synthetic cathinones and other stimulants. Additionally, over 1,000 kg of synthetic cannabinoids used to make herbal incense products and almost 800 kg of treated plant material were seized. This is by far the largest operation to date to target and interdict emerging drug distribution.

It is important to note that critics of the DEA's operations have argued that these large-scale efforts to bring down the manufacturing and distribution networks of gray markets run largely by business entrepreneurs may have the unintended consequences of driving production into black markets controlled by violent cartels and creating new problems. However, we have learned that not all emerging drugs permeate into the black market for a variety of reasons. There also is a lack of intelligence on what happens when the emerging drug trade shifts to black market distribution. For example, when mephedrone shifted to dealers in the UK, did these dealers acquire the product from distributors in the Far East with or without cartel influence? To be sure, if there is money to be made, traditional organized crime syndicates will find their way to exploit these opportunities. So, if not now, it is just a matter of time. Yet, there are substantial differences in the manufacture, distribution, and sales of these substances relative to their traditional illicit cousins.

For law enforcement, targeting the manufacturing and distribution of emerging drugs may be the most effective strategy. Local retail enforcement may be important given the large number of products that may still be on the shelves despite state and federal bans on these products. For example, the Chatham-Savannah Counter Narcotics Team (CNT) in Savannah, Georgia sent CNT officers to personally distribute letters to local gas stations and convenience stores advising them that synthetic marijuana products are dangerous and may contain controlled substances prior to the state and federal bans on these products taking effect. Although in some cases, operators of local convenience stores may not be aware of the legal status of these products, in this case, local law enforcement proactively notified local retail outlets. Despite these efforts, several arrests were made when undercover CNT agents were able to request and purchase herbal incense products that were being hidden under the counter (NACS 2012). This situation poses several questions for retailers who have left over products following a ban, including what to do with these products. In this case, the owner clearly knew these products were illegal and had removed them from the shelf, but still sold them to patrons who specifically requested them.

5.6 Prosecuting Emerging Drug Cases

Another major challenge of emerging drugs is in the prosecution of these cases, especially when the substance is not specifically scheduled. As discussed earlier, there is ambiguity in what is considered an "analogue" or being "substantially similar" to a controlled substance. A recent federal case in Arizona has successfully led to a conviction involving controlled substance analogues and will serve as a model to other jurisdictions in the future.

As part of the DEA operation "Log Jam," Michael Lane of Cave Creek, Arizona was arrested and found guilty of conspiracy to manufacture and distribute a controlled substance analogue and for possession with intent to distribute a controlled substance analogue (Lopez 2013). Lane worked and operated two businesses that marketed and sold bath-salt-type products. His product "Eight Ballz Bath Salts" contained MDPV, which was reformulated after the emergency scheduling of MDPV in October 2011. His new products including "Eight Ballz Ultra Premium Glass Cleaner," "Amped Lady Bug Attractant Exuberance Powder," "White Water Rapid Lady Bug Attractant Exuberance Powder," and "Snowman Glass Cleaner" contained the stimulants APVP (α-pyrrolidinopentiophenone), APBP (α-pyrrolidinobutiophenone), MPPP (desmethylprodine), and Pentedrone. These substances are similar to controlled substances and therefore the case was tried under the Federal Analogue Act.

Mr. Lane has yet to be sentenced, but the offense carries up to a 20-year sentence and a US$ 1 million fine. DEA Special Agent in Charge Doug Coleman stated "Friday's verdict serves notice to those who are contemplating entering this emerging area of the illegal drug industry" (as cited in Lopez 2013). This may signal the first in a series of cases targeting the manufacturing and distribution of emerging drugs and may effectively deter some of the reformulation of emerging drug products. Other federal cases are being tried in Minneapolis (regarding a Duluth case, see Karnowski 2013), South Dakota (in a town called Goodwin, see Hult 2013), among various others across the nation. Local courts may see an influx of similar cases, but evidence of this trend has not surfaced just yet. It is likely that many of these cases have been plead out by local prosecutors as taking these cases to trial are incredibly costly, primarily due to the forensic examination involved to help make the case.

5.7   Crime Lab and Drug Testing

While they are still in their legal gray market form, the primary appeal of novel drugs is that users can consume them with little fear of failing a drug test. Typically with novel substances, there is a lag between when a substance hits the market and the ability for drug tests to reliably detect the substance. Furthermore, it takes time for such innovation in drug testing technology to be put into practice in a uniform way. It is during this window of opportunity that these substances become particularly attractive to those who may be subjected to routine or even sporadic drug tests. This is especially the case for certain subpopulations subjected to frequent drug testing such as athletes, military personnel, and probationers (Stogner et al. 2012) among others (truck drivers, pilots, drug court participants, job applicants, etc.). For example, in response to the growing use of synthetic cannabinoids in the military, Army Col. Timothy Lyons, chief of toxicology in the Defense Department's medical examiner's office stated, "We have a difficulty detecting it" (as cited in Tilghman 2010) and has poured a vast amount of resources trying to remedy this issue.

This inability to test for controlled substances may also present challenges for law enforcement in that they must develop reliable and valid tests to identify these newly illicit substances. This creates a daunting task for crime laboratories and their forensic chemists who may be charged with trying to identify a large number of chemical compounds that might be contained in these products. David Murphy, acting assistant commissioner of the Office of Field Operations applauds the efforts of law enforcement chemists and outlines some of these challenges—"Additionally, I want to recognize the work of CBP scientists who have been instrumental in identifying synthetic drugs and identifying the new synthetic compounds that were created … they change one molecule, each time they change that a new test has to be created so this is hard work and this is great work and its very sophisticated work that our labs bring to the table" (Project Synergy Press Conference 2013). In each emerging drug case, analysts may be charged with developing and validating custom protocols to qualify the consistency of an unknown sample suspected of containing emerging drugs. This interrupts routinized identification of long-known illicit drugs which make up the vast majority of the submissions to a crime lab, putting a drain on resources manpower, and may require more expensive and more current instrumentation.

Forensic toxicologists have an easier time keeping up with the Joneses, per se. As new substances become banned, their metabolites can be quickly added to drug screens and scrutinized for in confirmatory tests. The sheer size of the drug testing industry in the USA almost ensures that the costs of these additions will be modest, at best as the demand for these more comprehensive tests expand. For the situations that call for increased scrutiny (e.g., DOT sensitive safety positions, drug court and treatment participants, community corrections, etc.), alternative types of monitoring can be utilized to ensure compliance. For example, random check-ins by supervisors or case managers may help, particularly in cases that have recently been flagged to drug test "for cause." The rules and restrictions should be readily apparent for individuals in these circumstances; that is, individuals should know what they are allowed to use (e.g., cigarettes and prescribed medication) and what they are not, including the substances not usually tested for. It may be the perception of many of these individuals that if we cannot test for it and it is not specifically illegal, then it is safe or clear use.

5.8   Emerging Drug Prevention

One way to address the growing concern over emerging drugs is through the use of educational campaigns. These campaigns have been designed to target those who are at highest risk for engaging in emerging drug use including teens, military members, and college students. Initially, because service members are often drug tested, some of the earliest reports of emerging drug use came from military sources, and, before statewide and federal bans on these products were issued, the military instituted its own policies prohibiting the use of these substances.

Among military personnel, emerging drugs present a unique challenge. Because service men and women are subjected to drug tests and even polygraphs about their drug use, traditional illicit drugs, although problematic, are often avoided. New "legal highs" present a problem among the armed forces since military personnel may seek out these substances as substitutes for illicit substances. Starting in 2005, the military became concerned with the use of salvia since it was not explicitly controlled under the Uniform Code of Military Justice (UCMJ). As a response, many military bases gave direct orders banning the use of salvia (Griffin et al. 2008).

As the use of salvia began to subside among armed services personnel, synthetic cannabinoids soon replaced it. The earliest problems started in 2008 when marine commanders had to issue a ban at one of their Japanese bases. During 2008 and 2009, the problem escalated with several airmen and soldiers caught with synthetic cannabinoids. The problem reached a precipice when the marine base commander at Camp Lejeune, NC, sent out letters to local stores asking them not to sell synthetic cannabinoids to marines. These events, along with a large-scale bust on the Japan-based aircraft carrier George Washington, led to the Navy issuing a service-wide ban (Tilghman 2010).

As a response to these problems, the pentagon began an "anti-spice" campaign (named after the popular brand of synthetic cannabinoids) starting in October 2010. On an October 1 broadcast on the Pentagon Channel, anchor marine staff Sgt. Josh Hauser stated, "One bad dose could cost you your life" (Tilghman 2010). On that same day, the American Forces Press Service published an article warning about the possible negative health outcomes of smoking synthetic marijuana. Several videos were soon released warning of the potential harm of these products and advising service members that they could be punished under the UCMJ for using them. The videos noted that there is a lot of uncertainty in what these products contain. For example, one video argued that marijuana is "the devil you know" and spice is "the devil you don't." Capt. Kevin Klette, a Navy doctor and head of the Department of Defense Drug Demand Reduction Program is quoted in the video saying, "You may one day have a bag that gives you the effect of normal marijuana. . . but then again you may have something that is 100 times more potent and could lead to death" (as cited in Tilghman 2010).

In December 2011, the Navy produced posters and ad campaigns for both "spice" and "bath salts." The slogan included for spice was "It's not legal. It's not healthy. It's not worth it." For bath salts the slogan was even more dramatic stating, "It's not a fad. . . . It's a nightmare" and included the depiction of a soldier looking into a mirror and a crazed zombie-like version of the individual looking back. In January 2013, the Navy released a six-and-a-half minute dramatized video depicting a bad bath salt "trip." The video is shot from a first-person perspective and is set to a "dubstep" track with anti-melodic rhythms and oscillating bass drops. First, the sailor receives bath salts in a package in the mail and snorts it. He then proceeds to vomit, steal food, have a violent encounter with his girlfriend, and hallucinate that his friend is a monster. Next, he collapses and is seen convulsing as medical personnel try to attend to him. The video then goes on to give information on how to recognize bath salts, how they are used, and the harms that they present including paranoid delusions, hallucinations, and even death.

The Department of Health of Washington, DC has adopted a similar strategy as the Navy. Although the primary focus of their campaign is on synthetic cannabinoids, they have extended the idea that emerging drugs are associated with "zombies." The ads that have recently debuted on the DC Metro depict teenagers dressed like zombies from a horror film. The teenage zombies are posed in various stages of decomposition with captions such as "No one wants to take a zombie to the prom" (DeBonis 2013). The campaign clarifies why they have associated synthetic cannabinoids with zombies stating, "Fake weed causes extreme anxiety, paranoia, panic attacks, alienation/disassociation, psychotic episodes, and hallucinations. This behavior has been labeled the 'zombie' effect" (as cited in DeBonis 2013). Critics of these campaigns have argued that these depictions of the drugs are gross exaggerations and have likened them to 1930s films like *Reefer Madness* (Sekaran 2013).

5.9 Future Directions

I want a new drug, one that won't make me sick. One that won't make me crash my car, or make me feel three feet thick. (Huey Lewis)

Moving forward, it will be important to build effective strategies to manage emerging drugs through a comprehensive, multidisciplinary effort. While many countries generally manage controlled substances in this manner by allowing medical expert testimony and hearing epidemiological evidence when deciding to schedule substances, we strongly believe that a branch of a regulatory agency should be dedicated to managing these products. This branch should consist of a diverse team of experts from conventional medicine, integrative medicine (which includes aspects of so-called alternative medicine but couched in empirical research), medicinal chemistry, pharmacy, epidemiology, and public policy. This expertise should address emerging psychoactive drugs as well as all products that have received the black box warning, "These statements have not been evaluated by the Food and Drug Administration. This product is not intended to diagnose, treat, cure, or prevent any disease."

Furthermore, nations and their media (the USA, in particular) are encouraged to veer away from the scare tactics it once used to keep individuals from thinking about using drugs. The most up-to-date and transparent information should emulate from institutions of authority in order to retain credibility with the population. Examples of recent embellishments or flat out unreliable reports regarding emerging drugs include: (1) the jenkem threat where users ferment feces and urine in a closed container and huff the resulting gases to get high (a desperate practice in some third world areas but extremely rare in modern nations), (2) the "krokodil" (clandestinely prepared desomorphine) threat that predicts this will be the next major drug craze in the USA to follow Russia's experience (a practice not likely emulated in nations with substantial supplies of powerful black market opiates/opioids), and (3) the salvia threat which would never surface primarily due to the lack of an appreciable continuance rate (e.g., the proportion of users that are likely to use again, suggestive of a substance's habit-forming nature). There needs to be some balanced effort to build a protocol that would enable a warning system which can better partition the emerging products that present an immediate and real threat to public health (such as bath salts) while avoiding the knee-jerk response of lumping all of these potential threats together (like trying to make the synthetic cannabinoids sound worse than they are with the zombie ads mentioned earlier).

Education materials need to be developed as soon as possible. It should be important to highlight the facts: we know little about the short-term effects of emerging drugs (particularly recently synthesized analogue products), we know even less about their long-term effects, and the fact that little scientific work is being done (or will be done) on the vast majority of these substances. Thus, these products are truly "use at your own risk."

As far as ramping up enforcement and compliance, we need to be mindful of particular segments of those that we closely monitor for drug use. Those who have DOT safety sensitive positions, who are engaged in treatment, participants in drug courts, or sentenced to community corrections all need clear parameters to set the right expectations. In regards to enforcement, local agencies may make progress by teaming up with those responsible for alcohol enforcement (typically state-level enforcers). These officials often visit convenience stores for compliance checks and to monitor sales to minors. As a part of their duties, the agents can educate owners about the risks in selling these products regardless of current legal status.

Last, we should acknowledge what we learn from drug using subcultures and apply it to our understanding of emerging drug trends. For example, emerging club drugs are likely to remain club drugs (e.g., the phenethylamines). The synthetic stimulants do not seem to be displacing the preference for cocaine, methamphetamine, and prescription stimulants. The only displacement seems to be in the club setting, particularly when MDMA supplies are low. Similarly synthetic marijuana seems to be tied to restricted personal access to marijuana. These understandings will allow us to focus efforts on reducing the harms to these segments through targeted efforts. In the end, by viewing emerging drugs individually, avoiding sensationalism, utilizing caution, and grounding policy in sound empirical research and careful deliberation, society can better sidestep the pitfalls associated with rampant use of new drugs or problematic legislation born out of a panic.

References

Americans for Safe Access. (2013). What's the cost?: The federal war on patients. A report on the casualties of the war on medical cannabis. June, 2013.
Blake, A. (2013, August 21). White House: Obama doesn't favor medical marijuana 'at this point.' *The Washington Post*. http://www.washingtonpost.com/blogs/post-politics/wp/2013/08/21/white-house-obama-doesnt-favor-medical-marijuana-at-this-point/ Accessed 27 Nov 2013.
Boos, T. (2011). Presentation on drug scheduling actions. 20th National Conference on Pharmaceutical and Chemical Diversion in Fort Worth, Texas. June 14-15, 2011.
Castellanos, D., Singh, S., Thornton, G., Avila, M., & Moreno, A. (2011). Synthetic cannabinoid use: A case series of adolescents. *Journal of Adolescent Health, 49*(4), 347–349.
DeBonis, M. (2013). City: 'Fake weed' will turn you into a zombie. *The Washington Post*. May 2, 2013. http://www.washingtonpost.com/blogs/mike-debonis/wp/2013/05/02/city-fake-weed-will-turn-you-into-a-zombie/
Drug Enforcement Administration (DEA). (2012). Nationwide synthetic drug takedown: 19 million packets of synthetic drugs seized and $36 million in cash. *DEA NEWS* July 26, 2012. http://www.justice.gov/dea/pubs/pressrel/pr072612.html Accessed 27 Nov 2013.
Drug Enforcement Administration (DEA). (2013). Updated results from DEA's largest-ever global synthetic drug takedown yesterday. *DEA NEWS* June 26, 2013. http://www.justice.gov/dea/divisions/hq/2013/hq062613.shtml Accessed 27 Nov 2013.
Federal Analogue Act of 1986. 21 U.S.C. § 813.
Florida House Bill 1363 (2008).
Goozner, M. (2004). *The $800 million pill: The truth behind the cost of new drugs*. University of California Press.
Griffin, O. H., III., Miller, B. L., & Khey, D. N. (2008). Legally high? Legal considerations of *Salvia divinorum. Journal of Psychoactive Drugs, 40*, 183–191.
Grinspoon vs. Drug Enforcement Administration, 828 F.2d 881 (1st Cir. 1987).
Hult, J. (2013). High court hears synthetic pot case. Argus Leader. http://www.argusleader.com/article/20131002/NEWS/310020051/High-court-hears-synthetic-pot-case
Indiana House Bill 1196 (2012). 117th General assembly, second regular session. http://www.in.gov/legislative/bills/2012/HE/HE1196.1.html
Iowa Senate Bill 2341 (2012). Appears to be 84th session. Yep - 84th general assembly. http://coolice.legis.iowa.gov/linc/84/external/SF2341_Introduced.pdf.
Jerry, J., Collins, G., & Streem, D. (2012). Synthetic legal intoxicating drugs: The emerging 'incense' and 'bath salt' phenomenon. *Cleveland Clinic Journal of Medicine, 79*, 258–264.

Johnson, K., & Chebium, R. (2013). Justice dept. won't challenge state marijuana laws. *USA Today*. August 29, 2013. http://www.usatoday.com/story/news/nation/2013/08/29/justice-medical-marijuana-laws/2727605/ Accessed 27 Nov 2013.

Karnowski, S. (2013). Guilty verdicts in Minnesota synthetic drugs case. Miami Herald. http://www.miamiherald.com/2013/10/07/3675868/guilty-verdict-in-minnesota-synthetics.html Accessed 27 Nov 2013.

Lopez, C. (2013). Federal jury convicts tempe designer drug maker/distributer on federal controlled substance analogue enforcement act violations. Press release. District of Arizona, The United States Attorney's Office. July 22, 2013. http://www.justice.gov/usao/az/press_releases/2013/PR_07222013_Lane.html Accessed 27 Nov 2013.

NACS. (2012). Georgia store busted for selling illegal substance. NACSonline. National Association of Convenience Stores. August 27, 2012. http://www.nacsonline.com/NACS/News/Daily/Pages/ND0827125.aspx

Project Synergy Press Conference (2013). U.S. Customs and Border Protection Office of Public [press release]. Affairs-Visual Communications Division. http://www.dvidshub.net/unit/USCBP#.UjC4SH-8BSo#ixzz2ebvWmohF Accessed 27 Nov 2013.

Pure Food and Drug Act. (1906). Pub. L. 59-386, 34 Stat. 768.

Sekaran, S. (2013). Synthetic marijuana turns people into zombies, says Atrocious govt. Anti-drug propaganda. *AlterNet*. May 14, 2013. http://www.alternet.org/drugs/synthetic-marijuana-turns-people-zombies-says-atrocious-govt-anti-drug-propaganda Accessed 27 Nov 2013.

Spillane, J. F. (2000). Cocaine: From medical marvel to modern menace in the United States, 1884-1920 (Vol. 18). JHU Press.

Stogner, J. M., Khey, D. N., Griffin, O. H., III., Miller, B. L., Boman, J. H., IV. (2012). Examining the effect of regulating a novel drug: An evaluation of changes in use of *Salvia divinorum* in the first year of Florida's ban. *International Journal of Drug Policy, 23*(6), 512–521.

Synthetic Drug Abuse Prevention Act. (2012). 21 U.S.C. § 811–812.

Tilghman, A. (2010). Pentagon launches anti-spice campaign. *NavyTimes*. October 14, 2010. http://www.navytimes.com/article/20101014/NEWS/10140345/Pentagon-launches-anti-spice-campaign Accessed 27 Nov 2013.

USA vs. Forbes, 806 F. Supp. 232, 1992.

Vandrey, R., W Johnson, M., S Johnson, P., & A Khalil, M. (2013). Novel drugs of abuse: A snapshot of an evolving marketplace. *Adolescent Psychiatry, 3*(2), 123–134.

Vardakou, I., Pistos, C., & Spiliopoulou, C. (2010). Spice drugs as a new trend: Mode of action, identification and legislation. *Toxicology letters, 197*(3), 157–162.

Wohlfarth, A., & Weinmann, W. (2010). Bioanalysis of new designer drugs. *Bioanalysis, 2*(5), 965–979.

Yeh, B. T. (2012). The Controlled Substance Act: Regulatory requirements. Congressional Research Service. CRS Report for Congress, 7-5700, RL34635

Index

A
Absinthe, 14–18
Adams, J., 15, 16
Adebamiro, A., 63
Agnew, R., 45
Ait-Daoud, N., 47
Akers, R.L., 23, 45
Albanese, A., 63
Albert, S., 68
Andreasen, M.A., 68
Angoa-Pérez, M., 7
Angrish, D., 62
Antonowicz, J.L., 63
Appel, J., 54
Arunotayanun, W., 3
Augsburger, M., 58
Auwärter, V., 46
Ayres, T.C., 5, 8, 40, 41

B
Bücheler, R., 56
Bachman, J.G., 7, 22, 46, 64
Baggott, M.J., 54
Baldacchino, A., 42
Barbanoj, M.J., 54
Barnett, T.E., 46
Baron, M., 8
Barratt, M.J., 40
Bath salts, 61–67
Baumann, M.H., 62
Beaver, K.M., 44
Becker, H., 45
Beuhler, M.C., 62, 64
Bird, S.B., 42
Birkler, R.I., 68
Black market, 38–41
Blake, A., 80
Boman, J., 45

Boman, J.H., 39, 45, 48
Bond, J.W., 5, 8, 40, 41
Boos, T., 85
Borna, C., 68
Botanical highs, 29
Bouso, J.C., 54
Boyd, C.J., 41
Boyer, E.W., 42
Brandt, S.D., 3, 63
Breathes, W., 30
Brewer, N.T., 42
Bromo-DragonFly, 68–70
Brush, D.E., 42
Burgess, R.L., 45

C
Cakic, V., 40
Camarasa, J., 7
Cantrell, F.L., 7
Carhart-Harris, R.L., 64, 66
Cary, P., 28
Castellanos, D., 84
Catbagan, P., 28
Caulkins, J.P., 9
Chandra, A., 59
Chebium, R., 80
Cicero, T.J., 41
Clapp, J.D., 59
Clark, R.F., 7
Cohen, P.A., 34
Cole, J., 63
Collins, G., 4
Cone, E.J., 5
Controlled Substance Act (CSA), 78,
    81, 83
Cook, R.L., 46
Coppola, M.M., 62, 63, 68
Corazza, O., 4, 8, 9, 63, 67–69
Corkery, J., 8, 63, 67

D. N. Khey et al., *Emerging Trends in Drug Use and Distribution*,
SpringerBriefs in Criminology 12, DOI 10.1007/978-3-319-03575-8,
© Springer International Publishing Switzerland 2014

Coulson, C., 9
Courtwright, D.T., 14
Crichlow, V.J., 45
Cross, J., 66
Cunningham, J.A., 43
Cupps, S., 59
Curran, H.V., 63

D
Dabbing, 29, 30
Dahl, J., 65
Dang, Q., 47
Daniel, J., 59
Dargan, P.I., 5, 47, 63, 68
Davey, Z., 8, 67
Davies, S., 3, 40, 41
de Jager, A.D., 28
DeBonis, M., 90
Deluca, P., 8, 42, 67
Dennehy, C.E., 41, 55, 58
Designer drugs, 4
Detrick, B., 1
Dickerson, T.J., 62
Dillon, N., 1
Dresen, S., 46
Drug
    analogues, 78, 87
    distribution, 33, 37, 38
    history, 13, 14, 25
    information, 43, 45
    manufacturing, 37
    panic, 2, 9
    prevalence, 57, 68
    prevention, 89, 90
    regulation, 9, 10
    scare, 25, 26, 30
    testing, 88, 89
    trends, 26–30
    use, 57, 60, 64, 67
Dunn, K.E., 46
Dybdal-Hargreaves, N.F., 6, 8, 62

E
Earls, F., 46
Emerging drugs, 1, 2, 6–9
    definition, 3–5
    sources, 5, 6
    use, 8, 33–38, 43–48
Erickson, T., 66
Erowid, E., 54
Erowid, F., 54
Escher. Mephedrone, C., 63
Escubedo, E., 7

F
Fass, A.D., 46, 62
Fass, J.A., 5, 46, 62–64
Felber, F., 58
Fergus, S., 63
Ferguson, W., 28
Ferreirós, N., 46
Festinger, D.S., 43, 58
Fischer, R.G., 28
Flanagin, A.J., 42
Forman, R.F., 43, 58
Francescutti, D.M., 7
Freeman, S., 63
Freeman, T.P., 63
Fry, J.A., 46

G
Gaertner, I., 56
Gajagowni, R.G., 67
Gallegos, A.N.A., 38
Garcia, A.S., 46, 62
Ghodse, A.H., 63
Gibbons, S., 3
Ginsburg, B.C., 36
Girling, E.R., 46
Giroud, C., 58
Gleiter, C.H., 56
Goda, Y., 40
Goldberger, B., 62
González, D., 54, 60
Goode, E., 44
Goozner, M., 79
Gordon, R.A., 44
Gottfredson, M.R., 45
Gómez-Jarabo, G., 54
Green, N., 65
Grey market, 41
Griffin, O.H., 1, 13, 38, 45, 55, 56,
    80, 89
Griffiths, P., 38
Gunderson, E., 47
Gustavsson, D., 63

H
Hall, A., 28
Halpern, J.H., 28
Hart, C., 47
Haugen, L.S.Y., 63
Haughey, H., 47
Helgesen, R.D., 28
Hendricks, L., 47
Henman, M., 28
Hiaasesn, S., 65

Hibberd, P.L., 42
Hirschi, T., 45
Hofmann, A., 18
Holder, N.D., 62
Homer, K., 59
Hoover, V., 43, 58
Horisberger, B., 58
Hosanagar, A., 62
Hu, X., 46
Hult, J., 87
Hulten, P., 68
Humphreys, K.N., 43
Hussain, N., 63

I
Inciardi, J.A., 22, 41
International drug distribution, 37, 38
International drug law, 84
Internet, 55, 58, 59, 62, 68
Iverson, R.B., 67

J
Jansen, J., 7, 46, 62
Javors, M.A., 36
Jerry, J., 4, 5, 83
Johannsen, M., 68
Johnson, G., 64
Johnson, K., 80
Johnson, T.J., 42
Johnston, L.D., 7, 22, 46, 64
Joshi, A., 47
Junge, T., 62

K
Kane, M.J., 7
Karila, L., 64
Karimi, K., 63
Karnowski, S., 87
Kawahara, N., 40
Kaye, B.K., 42
Kempton, R.J., 22
Kempton, T., 22
Khan, S., 62
Khey, D.N., 1, 38, 40, 41, 43,
    45, 55, 56
Kikura-Hanajiri, R., 40
Kim-Appel, D., 54
Kratom, 82
Kriikku, P., 63
Krohn, M.D., 45
Kuhn, D.M., 7
Kurtz, S.P., 41
Kyle, P.B., 67
Kypri, K., 43

L
Lachenmeier, D.W., 15
Lange, J.E., 59
Lee, J., 69
Lee, M.A., 14
Legal highs, 3–5, 7
Lenton, S., 40
Lopez, C., 87
Lopez, D., 38
Lucaites, V.L., 35
Lysergic acid diethylamine (LSD), 18–21

M
3,4-methylenedioxymethamphetamine
    (MDMA), 23, 24, 27
Müller, M., 46
Mangin, P., 58
Marlowe, D.B., 43, 58
Marona-Lewicka, D., 35
Marsden, J., 5, 63
Martínez-Clemente, J., 7
Massey, J.L., 45
Maurer, H.H., 63
McAulifre, W.E., 44
McCabe, S.E., 41
McElrath, K., 39, 63, 66
McMahon, L.R., 36
McNamara, S., 63
Measham, F., 47, 63
Media coverage, 55, 68, 69
Medical marijuana, 80
Mendelson, J.E., 54
Methylenedioxypyrovalerone (MDPV),
    62–66
Metzger, A.K., 63
Metzger, M.J., 42
Meyer, M.R., 63
Miller, A.E., 41, 55, 58
Miller, B.L., 1, 4, 38, 39, 45, 48,
    55, 56, 64
Miller, J.M., 4
Mitcheson, L., 5, 63
Mohammed, A.M., 7
Molina, J., 62
Mondola, R.R., 62, 63, 68
Moore, C., 28
Moore, K., 47
Morgan, C.J., 63
Morris, H., 27
Murphy, C.M., 62, 64
Murray, B.L., 62–64
Mushtaq, S., 62

N
Nakajima, J.I., 40
Natural highs, 29
Natural medicinal products, 28
Nelson, D.L., 35
Nelson, S., 62, 63, 65
Nichol, D.E, 35
Nicholson, K.L., 7
Nielsen, V.T., 68
Novak, S.J., 19
Novel drug marketing, 38–41

O
O'Malley, P.M., 7, 22, 46, 64
O'Neill, C., 39, 63, 66
Online drug sales, 40, 41
Ottoson, P.E., 62

P
Pütz, M., 46
Parker, M.A., 35
Patapis, N.S., 43, 58
Patočka, J., 15
Pavarin, R.M., 58
Peltoniemi, T., 42
Perazella, M.A., 63
Perrone, D., 28
Personne, M., 68
Peters, F.T., 63
Pistos, C., 36
Plucar, B., 15
Pope, H.G., 28
Porrovecchio, A., 64
Pratt, T.C., 45
Primack, B.A., 46
Prisinzano, T.E., 54
Prosser, L.M., 62, 63
Pubill, D., 7
Public health, 2–4, 10
    concerns, 7–9

Q
Quaalude, 21–23

R
Ramanujam, S.L., 63
Rana, S., 28
Raudenbush, S.W., 46
Ray, O., 22
Reed, M.B., 59
Regulating drugs, 75, 76
Reynaud, M., 64
Riba, J., 54
Rivier, L., 58

Rodrigues, W.C., 28
Roff, A.N., 66
Rome, J., 65
Rosner, P., 62
Ross, E.A., 62
Ryan, M.L., 7, 46, 62

S
Salvia, 53–58
Salvia divinorum, 53–61, 80–83
Sampson, R.J., 46
Sanchez, J.J., 36
Santonastaso, P., 8, 67
Sarwar, H., 62
Scherbaum, N., 42
Schifano, F., 8, 42, 63, 67
Schulenberg, J.E., 7, 46, 64
Schumacher, B., 68
Schuster, F., 62
Schwoerer, P., 56
Sedefov, R., 38
Seefeld, A., 7
Sekaran, S., 90
Selby, P.L., 43
Seto, T., 40
Shadow industry, 33–36
Shah, M.M., 7
Shaheen, F., 62
Shannon, M., 42
Sheridan, M., 65
Shulgin, A., 27
Simonato, P., 8, 67
Singleton, M., 4
Skinner, W.F., 45
Smith, A., 27
Smith, T.R., 45
Sonnichsen, F., 62
Spencer, L., 67
Spiliopoulou, C., 36
Spillane, J.F., 78
Spiller, H.A., 7, 9, 46, 62, 64
Spring, T., 55
Stair, J.L., 63
State drug laws, 75, 79
Stern, N., 62
Stogner, J.M., 4, 39, 41, 44–46, 48, 56,
    59, 64, 81, 82, 88
Streem, D., 4
Streur, W.J., 63
Sumnall, H.R., 5, 63
Surratt, H.L., 41
Suzuki, J., 40
Sweeney, M.D., 62

Sykes, K.E., 7
Synthetic cathinones, 65, 66, 69
Synthetic Drug Abuse Prevention Act, 77,
    83, 84
Synthetic drugs, 4, 27, 28
Synthetic legal intoxicating drugs (SLIDs), 4
Synthetic stimulants, 61

T
Taffe, M.A., 62
Takahashi, M., 40
Telving, R., 68
Thorlacius, K., 68
Tilghman, A., 88–90
Torrens, M., 42
Tsourounis, C., 41, 55, 58

U
U.S. drug law, 79, 80
Uchiyama, N., 40, 41

V
Vandewater, S.A., 62
Vandrey, R., 6, 46, 47
Vardakou, I., 4, 36, 37, 83, 84
Vaughn-Jones, J., 63
Vohra, R., 7

W
Wang, G., 28
Warner, J.V., 28
Warr, M., 45
Wasson, R.G., 54
Watson, M., 62
Way, W.L., 23
Weil, A.T., 13, 20
Weinmann, W., 46
Weston, R.G., 7, 46, 62
Westphal, F., 62
Wiley, J.L., 35
Wilhelm, J., 63
Williams, T., 62
Winder, G.S., 62, 63
Winstock, A.R., 5, 39, 63, 66
Wojcieszak, J., 54
Wood, D.M., 47, 68
Wright, M., 23
Wright, M.J. Jr., 62

Y
Yeh, B.T., 76, 77

Z
Zawilska, J.B., 54
Zwarun, L., 42

DATE DUE	RETURNED

CPSIA information can be obtained at www.ICGtesting.com
Printed in the USA
LVOW05s0745251014

410481LV00004B/49/P